THE PALEO DIET COOKBOOK FOR BEGINNERS

The Healthy Way of Living

FREE BONUS INCLUDED!

Tanya Simons

Kelly My friend
227
2891

Margarette
v 483 505
2902

Introduction

I want to thank you and congratulate you for purchasing the book, *"The ultimate Paleo Diet Cook book for beginners"*.

This book contains proven steps and strategies on how to live a healthy life and lose weight.

Thanks again for purchasing this book, I hope you enjoy it!

In order to grab your **FREE BONUS**

Please visit

https://infinitypublishers.leadpages.co/paleo-diet-web-page-/

Also if you gain any value from this book, please take the time **to share your thoughts and post a review on Amazon.** It'd be greatly appreciated!

Thank you.

Tanya Simons

Table of Contents

INTRODUCTION

You may know of people who must consume specific cakes or cookies every day. Such people are usually frowned upon as more often than not, they complain about the size of their body but they can't seem to shake off the desire to indulge in unhealthy foods. Research is still going on about this issue but so far, some progress has been made. This is focused on grains containing gluten. Gluten proteins are reduced to form peptides, which are able to stimulate opioid receptors (these are found in the brain and are usually stimulated by the likes of heroin and also when we do intense activities like running.)

Though research is still going on, I can testify to craving for pastry until I stopped consuming grains. Now you know if you are addicted to some grain product or know someone who is, just take grains off your diet and watch what happens!

Let's delve into a little science; grains have a lot of carbohydrates. Once they enter your digestive system, they undergo a process that turns them into glucose. This is used to fuel the body as you perform various activities that use up energy. Any glucose not used is stored as fat to be used in the future in case the body is not able to access food or when our bodies use a lot of energy. Our bodies are wired like this to ensure survival even in the harshest of conditions. Fortunately or unfortunately, most people can easily access food. The result is large stores of fat in the body. This is what eventually leads to obesity as well as hormonal roller coasters.

The bottom line is, our ancestors, the cavemen did not eat grains and all this junk we have today. As a result, they had bodies to die for! They were smart enough to know that the human body was not made for grains. After the agricultural revolution, grains were consumed but not in such high amounts as we see today. Processed products such as flour could only be afforded by the rich, probably the reason why they died earlier than the common man. No one can argue with the fact that in the last century of increased grain consumption, the human population has recorded the highest number of obese people, high infertility rates and a very huge number of chronic diseases. Research conducted by the University of Missouri has found an inverse relationship between grain consumption and the testicular size. Additionally, they found that the sperm count of the average American male has dropped by 50% in the last eighty years!

 In as much as there are no immediate effects witnessed in the consumption of grains, especially, whole grains; this does not give us the clear sign to indulge in grains; bearing in mind that the consumption of grains today is at its all-time high.

It all boils down to this; if you treat your body like a temple, you will shine in the glory of its beauty. Grains were not made for our bodies. It's as simple as that. With the case of whole grains and refined grain, it is like saying take cigarettes that have got filters and avoid those without filters. At the end of the day cigarettes are bad for your health and you should avoid them at all costs! So it is with grains; pasta, rice, cookies, bread, to name but a few. They should all be scraped off from our diets.

Conduct a small experiment to judge for yourself. Take a week off from anything that spells out the word grain and see just how much energy you will have. Increase your intake of vegetables and fruits and I can guarantee not only will your energy levels soar through the roof but you will have gone more than a mile in shedding some of that unwanted body fat. Why not go the extra mile and eliminate grains from your diet?

If you want to get a better body, you know exactly what to do!

WHAT IS A PALEO APPROACH?

A Paleo approach allows fruits, veggies, nuts, seeds, seafood and meats and does not allow grains, legumes, dairy, selected vegetable oils such as corn oil, soy oil and cotton seed oil. Starchy vegetables such as tubers lie in a gray area as there are some Paleo followers who eat them while there are

Collard greens, kale and almonds (you can even make almond milk to substitute for dairy milk. Additionally, the Paleo approach emphasizes on non-starchy veggies and lean meats making it very different from other low carb meal plans that usually include too much fat and very little protein and veggies.

You will be surprised to learn that an estimated 50 million Americans live with some form of autoimmune condition. Yeah, that's some who do not.

You have probably stumbled on some information claiming that the Paleo approach may contain too much fat and not enough fiber, vitamin D and calcium. I respectfully disagree with these concerns as all these are things that can be addressed. For one, vegetables provide protein, fiber, calcium, and vitamin D, which are usually obtained from dairy foods. They can be gotten by increasing your consumption of broccoli, right! Well, if you are among this number you know all too well that in as much as modern medicine is hyped, it really doesn't do much to alleviate your condition. It's not time to give up hope as you will learn with the Paleo & gluten free approach.

To start with, the paleo approach bans certain foods that are continually marketed as 'healthy' like soy, whole grains and low-fat dairy. The main reason for this is that these foods are the major culprits behind various autoimmune conditions. This approach cleanses your body, calms your immune system, resolves all inflammation problems, and helps your body heal itself.

The renowned philosopher Hippocrates discovered the healing

power of food and the importance of feeding our bodies with natural and nutritious foods. He said, "Let they food be thy medicine and thy medicine be thy food." Remember the garbage in garbage out principle? It's the same thing only that Hippocrates additionally discovered that if you feed your body with pure, natural, and whole foods, your body will have no single reason to complain.

A major concern for most people about embracing the Paleo diet is that this approach will break the bank or even take too much of your time. This is one hundred percent not true! It might have been true back then when the approach was just starting out, but today, there are so many places where you can find fresh fruits and veggies and grass-fed beef among other foods that are supported by the Paleo approach such as the farmer's market and selected food stores. Later on I will be sharing with you a few recipes just to give you an idea of how easy and pocket friendly it is to prepare Paleo foods; together with a two-week meal plan to help you get the most out of your food.

What to Expect When You Embrace a Paleo Diet

Let' start by delving into a bit of history just to help you get a glimpse of what is the store for you. Millions and millions of year ago, human being fed on wild plant and animals –this is a paleo diet. And about ten thousand year ago, people embraced a totally different way of eating a grain cultivation was adopted. This caused a huge shock to our system as we were forced to shift from our evolutionary diet of fresh fruits, vegetables, and animal products to a diet characterized by lots of grains and legumes.

Comparing 10,000 years with millions of years, it is approximately months if not weeks of a 40 year old person's life. This implies that our bodies have got very little time to adjust to this way of eating. Again, comparing the condition of our bodies millions of years ago (during the Paleolithic era) with our bodies now (after the agricultural revolution), based on archeological evidence, our Paleolithic bodies were disease free and muscular compared to the fat and disease ridden bodies of today.

Even up to date, our bodies are still adept at eating what our ancestors ate and adopting a paleo diet is going to immensely benefit you. However, I'm going to be honest with you; shifting from the little-nutrition, high-energy standard Western diet to a high-fat and –fiber, low-carb Paleo diet won't be easy for your system to adapt, which is very normal.

First, when starting the paleo diet, your body will be detoxified to eliminate all toxins and waste products that have accumulated in your body courtesy of eating highly processed and refined foods that are loaded with preservatives, flavorings, colorings, and other harmful chemicals. And as with any form of detoxification, you might experience cravings, dizziness, nausea, diarrhea or constipation, weakness and headaches. Fortunately, all these side effects will go away with time.

Why paleo?

As aforementioned, human beings have been feeding on fruits, vegetables, meat, nuts and seed for about 99.5% of our time on earth. For the remaining 0.5% (since farming began), we have been eating legumes and grains. Clearly, our bodies have not adapted to eating such foods, not to mention the refined and processed versions lined on shelves of supermarkets and food stores today.

This drastic change in our eating lifestyle is at the root of the degenerative diseases such as diabetes, obesity, cancer, depression, high blood pressure, heart disease, Alzheimer's disease, Parkinson's disease, and infertility. Shifting back to eating what our ancestors ate thousands of years ago, we eradicate the foods that are at odds with our bodies and also increase our consumption of antioxidants, vitamins and minerals.

NOTE: If have any health issues or you're on medication, please check with your physician to see if you are fit to embrace the Paleo approach before starting on the diet.

Paleo diet Food List

For a quick 'eat' and 'don't eat' paleo, here is a quick reference guide:

Eat	Don't Eat
Fresh fruits	Dairy
Fresh vegetables	Legumes (including legumes)
Seafood/fish	Cereal grains
Grass-fed meats	Potatoes
Free-range eggs	Refined sugar
Nuts	Salty foods
Seeds	Processed foods
Healthy oils such as coconut, extra virgin olive oil, macadamia, flaxseed, walnut, and avocado	Cereal grains
	Refined vegetable oils

The Paleo Diet Meats

This is a list of all the meats you can enjoy when following a paleo diet. The good thing is that almost all the meats are paleo. But remember to stay away from the highly processed meats and meat products such as hot dogs, spam, and other low quality, high-fat meats.

- Chicken livers
- Pork loin
- Duck
- Goat meat
- Lean hamburger
- Chuck Steak
- Lean Beef
- Flank Steak
- Lean chicken breast
- Pork Chops
- Turkey breast
- Goose
- Lean poultry
- Lean Pork Trimmed
- Top Sirloin Steak
- Lean veal
- Rabbit meat
- Organ meats of chicken, beef, pork and lamb

Paleo Diet Fish and Seafood

All fish are on the paleo diet and they are loaded with good stuff like omega-3 fatty acids as well. Rule of thumb is if it has fins and swims, it is definitely paleo! Enjoy it!

- Scrod
- Shrimp
- Tuna
- Scallops
- Crab
- Herring
- Flatfish
- Red snapper
- Crayfish
- Grouper
- Lobster
- Monkfish
- Perch
- Halibut
- Mackerel
- Northern Pike
- Salmon
- Trout
- Mussels
- Rockfish
- Turbot

- Drum
- Oysters
- Shark

Paleo diet Nuts and Seeds

- Pecans
- Almonds
- Hazelnuts
- Walnuts
- Pumpkin Seeds
- Sunflower Seeds
- Brazil Nuts
- Macadamia Nuts
- Pistachios (unsalted)
- Cashews
- Sesame Seeds
- Chestnuts
- Pine Nuts

Paleo Diet Vegetables

Almost all veggies are paleo. However, the high-starch vegetables, such as squashes and potatoes have low nutritional value compared to the amount of carbs/sugars/starches they contain. While you might have them, they aren't always good for your health.

- Watercress
- Swiss Chard
- Radish
- Turnips
- Asparagus
- Tomato
- Lettuce
- Bell Peppers
- Peppers
- Turnip Greens
- Kohlrabi
- Spinach
- Dandelion
- Seaweed
- Onions
- Parsnip
- Mustard Greens
- Pumpkin
- Cauliflower
- Parsley
- Cabbage
- Green Onions
- Mushrooms
- Kale

- Celery
- Broccoli
- Eggplant
- Collards
- Brussels Sprouts
- Cucumber
- Artichoke
- Carrots

Eat these veggies in moderation as they are quite starchy.

- Yam
- Acorn squash
- Butternut squash
- Beets
- Sweet potatoes

Paleo Diet Oils/Fats

Many people believe that fat makes you fat; this is not true. Carbs do. Healthy fats and oils are a great source of creating energy. Here are some of the healthy paleo oils and fats.

- Olive oil (I prefer extra virgin olive oil)
- Coconut oil
- Avocado oil
- Macadamia oil

Paleo Diet Nuts

Everyone loves nuts and they are paleo. However, you need to be careful as cashews are high in fat, and they are very addictive —you can easily consume an entire jar in one sitting! If losing weight is your primary goal of adopting paleo diet, limit the amount of nuts you consume.

- Pecans
- Almonds
- Hazelnuts
- Walnuts
- Pumpkin Seeds
- Sunflower Seeds
- Brazil Nuts
- Macadamia Nuts
- Pistachios (unsalted)
- Cashews
- Sesame Seeds
- Chestnuts
- Pine Nuts

Note: Peanuts are not nuts and they aren't paleo either. They are a legume!

Paleo Diet Fruits

Fruits are delicious and very nutritious too. However, even the paleo approved fruits, contain fructose in large amounts, which, while much better than the high-fructose corn syrup (HFCS), is still sugar. Therefore, if your goal for adopting the paleo approach is to lose weight, you will want to cut back on the amount of fruits you consume and instead indulge more on the paleo-friendly veggies. That said; feel free to take one to three servings of fruit per day.

- Avocado

- Apple

- Blackberries

- Blueberries

- Plums

- Papaya

- Peaches

- Grapes

- Mango

- Lychee

- Orange

- Lemon

- Lime

- Tangerine

- Cantaloupe

- Raspberries

- Strawberries

- Guava
- Watermelon
- Pineapple
- Bananas
- Figs

Note: Consume high-sugar fruits in moderation.

Spices and Herbs

- Cinnamon
- Caraway
- Bay leaves
- Arise
- Basil
- Celery seeds
- Cayenne pepper
- Chivalry
- Ginger
- Garlic
- Chives
- Cilantro
- Coriander
- Clove
- Cumin

- Curry
- Dill
- Fenugreek
- Fennel
- Horseradish
- Juniper berry
- Lavender
- Rosemary
- Lemongrass
- Mint
- Marjoram
- Wasabi
- Vanilla
- Turmeric
- Tarragon
- Thyme
- Black pepper
- Peppermint
- Parsley
- Paprika
- Oregano
- Mustard

Foods to Avoid

When following paleo diet, you should avoid all refined and processed foods, sugar, legumes, and grains (especially gluten).

Dairy

For a strict paleo diet, we suggest you avoid all diaries. But if you choose it, we recommend that it be organic and raw. Avoid following Diary Products.

- Milk
- Yogurt
- Kefir
- Butter
- Buttermilk
- Cream
- Cottage cheese
- Dairy spreads
- Ice cream
- And everything from animal's teat

Soft drinks

All soft drinks, Coke, and pop contain high amounts of sugar and are not Paleo.

Fruit Juices

Avoid all canned fruit juices as they are super high in sugar. Instead extract your own fresh juice from fresh fruits such as oranges, limes, lemon, pineapple, etc.

Grains

Stay away from anything that contains a grain in it.

Legumes

Unfortunately, all legumes are not paleo. Here are legumes you should avoid:

All beans

- Kidney beans
- Horse beans
- Garbanzo beans
- Fava beans
- Broad beans
- Black beans
- White beans
- Red beans
- Pinto beans
- Navy beans
- Adzuki beans
- Mung beans
- Lima beans
- String beans
- Green beans

Peas

- Sugar snap peas
- Snow peas
- Chickpeas
- Black-eyed peas (and, yes, you should also avoid the

band)

Lentils

Miso

Peanuts

Peanut butter

Soybeans

Mesquite

Lupines

Tofu

Artificial Sweeteners

Unfortunately all sweeteners are not paleo, sweetie. In fact, by definition, they are artificial and not paleo. Always use honey or maple syrup to sweeten your food.

Salty Foods

Stay away from all overly salty foods because they are not paleo.

- Ketchup
- French fries

What should I drink on Paleo?

While water is considered the best natural hydrator, the paleo diet also offers options of other healthy beverages. Here are the paleo beverage options you can choose from and others you should avoid at all costs:

Water

Water, the prime hydrator, satisfies you as no other drink does. Pure water is chemical and toxin free has no artificial additives of any kind and is the only drink our ancestors relied on for maximum hydration. You need water for all kinds of bodily functions and overall good health; it's definitely the beverage of choice for those on a paleo diet. And regardless of the amount you drink there's no cause for concern concerning caloric intake. You may want to squeeze in a dash of lime or lemon juice to make plain water more exciting.

Herbal Teas

All types of natural herbal tea made by steeping health infused herbs into water provide a great way of staying hydrated while on a paleo diet. These natural herbal infusions offer a variety of aromas and tastes to enjoy and can also be found in non-caffeine varieties. The most common herbal teas include peppermint, ginger, nettle, green tea, and chamomile to name a few.

Fruit Juice

Store bought fruit juice usually comes with added sugar and preservatives. Unless it's 100% juice that contains no added ingredients, commercially prepared fruit juice isn't a healthy beverage on the paleo diet. It is better to eat fresh fruit instead of the packaged juice which is also devoid of fiber and other important nutrients.

Coffee and Tea

Caffeinated beverages normally stimulate cravings that come from blood sugar level imbalances. With fluctuating blood sugar, these drinks play an important role in keeping you going through the day. However, such urges and needs tend to be experienced by people who don't have enough nutritional intakes. Paleo diet followers normally get their fill from the nutrient dense foods high in fiber, fat and protein and don't need caffeinated beverages to perk them up. If the urge for caffeinated drinks seems hard to suppress, an occasional coffee without sugar and milk or black tea may be tolerated.

Milk

Milk and other dairy products are normally a no-no on a paleo eating plan. However, some versions, which are slightly lenient, make allowances for minimal dairy intake. Here only unpasteurized milk, preferably raw, is recommended.

Alcohol

The majority of paleo diet versions support an occasional drink or so. The trick here, however, is moderation and if moderation drinking is not possible with you, then maybe abstention may be your best course. Among alcohol, wine is the most recommended as it's made from fermented grapes as opposed to others that are derived from grains instead. Research indicates that consuming bear and other ales may cause similar effects as consuming grain based foods. Alcoholic drinks such as mead and tequila are considered better options as they are not made from grains.

Sodas and Other Sweet / Diet Beverages

Packed with chemicals and flavorings, artificial dyes, and refined sugars, these otherwise popular beverages are a total no-no from the get go. Beverages that contain artificial sweeteners include other synthetic chemicals that cause many health concerns. And artificial sweeteners only increase sugar craving which is not healthy. The only instance that the sports drinks can be allowed on a paleo diet is when the high endurance athletes are carrying out an intense training and are in need of electrolytes to replenish fluid loss fast.

The Health Benefits of a Paleo Approach

Let's have a look at some of the reasons you should waste no time to embracing the paleo approach. Nutrition has always been a subject very close to my heart and something has been bothering me for quite some time. When walking down the street or when going hopping to a supermarket, what is the first thing you notice? For me, it's the ever-increasing number of obese and overweight people (adults and kids alike) strolling down the street, and even worse, the food choices they make in the supermarkets.

True, everyone knows that processed foods should be avoided at all cost, physical activities should be carried out at least three times a week, and so on; but even with all this knowledge, the 'America the great' is the fattest country! I think mindless eating habits are to blame for all the health issues we are experiencing. And that is the reason why I'm an advent follower of the healthy paleo diet.

This diet goes to the very root of why we need food. Back in the hunter-gatherers' time, life was very simple (depending on how you look at it). During those days, men would go hunting very early in the morning while women would go gather fresh fruits, vegetables, nuts, and seeds. They would then come back home, cook, eat, and then relax, waiting for the next day, where the process would start again.

☐   Physical exercise –check

☐   Exposure to the sun – check

☐   Healthy and nutritious food – check

☐   Adequate sleep – check

Today, all these things have become so elusive that not even kids can achieve them. With a bank loan to pay, a mortgage, your children's college fees, and so on, it's almost impossible to even sleep –everyone is spending all of their time looking for more and more money. But the question is of what use is the money when you burn out and spend all the cash earned to pay the hospital bill?

With the paleo approach, your health is your first priority; everything else can wait. If you're a mother, you're going to be even a better mother when your health is at its best.

The Paleo diet isn't just a diet, it is a lifestyle change that primarily focus on achieving the four things I aforementioned above. By adequate sleep, I mean sleeping for 8 hours at the very minimum. Nutritious foods are all the foods contained on the paleo diet food list (think of wholefoods – fresh fruit, veggies, nuts, seeds, and everything our forefathers ate or drunk). Towards the end I will share with you healthy paleo recipes along with an amazing meal plan that will help ease you into the Paleo approach not forgetting mindful eating.

Now back to basics – the benefits of the Paleo diet. I had mentioned before that the paleo diet is one of the healthiest and most effective tools for losing weight. There are many weight loss programs, plans, and diet out there that promise to work wonders. So, what makes the Paleo approach so special?

First, most of the fad weight loss diets that exist today expose you to a high risk of developing some health problems and they can easily land you on a hospital bed. With these diets, you will lose weight very fast, and this is a problem in itself. And others are just hoaxes that will only help you lose the 'water weight' and after a few weeks, all the lost weight is back!

Now, let's look at the reasons that make the paleo diet to be in its own league:

☐　It doesn't ask you to take in unhealthy foods. The approach advocates for wholefoods and the unhealthy stuff does not make the cut in this diet.

☐　It doesn't advocate for extreme procedures, such as intense detoxification and cleansing – the diet itself is enough detox and cleanse.

☐   Food restrictions and fasting are not part of the approach.

☐   No counting calories or limiting the food intake

Prevention and Reduction of Chronic Disorders Symptoms

The paleo diet offers countless health benefit thanks to its natural and pure foods. The approach prevents arthritis, multiple sclerosis, celiac disease, heart disease, Alzheimer's disease, Crohn's disease, IBS, and much more. In addition to the prevention of these diseases, the paleo approach reduces the symptoms of patients suffering from these diseases.

No Bloating!

The paleo diet is rich in fiber, and when you combine this with low sodium intake and regular water intake, you have the ultimate recipe for reducing bloating that is very common, especially with the Western diet. The good thing about paleo diet is that it promotes microbiomes (healthy gut flora); thereby maintain a clean and healthy digestive system.

Detoxification

The paleo diet is all about consuming whole and real foods – save for a few condiment and bottled sauces. This means that you've completely eliminated hidden sugars, artificial flavorings, preservatives, colorings, hidden fats, you name it. Consequently, you fill up your system with healthy nutrients and eliminate all harmful toxins and chemicals from your body.

Healthy And Sustainable Weight Loss

Every paleo follower has experienced a massive weight loss, and the diet helps them maintain their new and healthy weight. Our forefathers used to have lean, healthy bodies, right? This is because the diet promotes muscle growth, better sleep, improved metabolic processes, sufficient vitamin D, gut health, good supply of omega-3/6 fatty acids, and better stress management –all of which play an important role in burning off excess body fat.

Increased nutrient intake

With the paleo diet, you'll eliminate processed carbs (what I usually refer to as the fillers) that actually have zero nutrition. Such foods are replaced by fresh fruits, vegetables, healthy fats, seeds and nuts, which are loaded with essential nutrients. With a healthy gut (that the diet promotes), you have an improved nutrient absorption .This is the reason why you'll notice all paleo diet followers have strong nails, glowing skin, and luscious locks – when your inside is healthy, it how on your outside!

Promotion of a Healthy Gastrointestinal System

The paleo diet advocates for the consumption of lots and lots of fresh fruits and veggies, which are rich sources of dietary fiber and other nutrients and minerals. The consumption of adequate amounts of fiber is linked to the reduction of constipation, hemorrhoids, rectal cancer, fissures and colon cancer.

Resolves Reproduction Problems

If you're a health enthusiast, like me, you've probably noticed the increased cases of infertility and reproductive problems. The reason behind this is that our diet is laden with harmful chemicals (especially the preservatives). Most of these chemicals we consume have similar characteristics with the hormone estrogen. So when these chemicals get in human system, they mimic the hormone estrogen and consequently cause reproductive problems. If you ask the expert, and even according to my thinking, this is why many men, today, have boobs (or mobs –as they are popularly referred to)

The paleo diet starts by cleansing and detoxifying your system. This process rids your body of these chemicals, toxins and other intruders that may be in your system and this is a big step in improving fertility.

Acne Fighter

Many researchers have spent sleepless nights trying to find out what causes acne. We used to believe that acne was caused by a bacterial infection but researchers later unveiled these four causes:

- ☐   Food allergies

- ☐   Insulin resistance

- ☐   Poor gut flora

- ☐   Hormonal imbalance

The paleo diet helps solve each of these four issues, leaving you with an acne-free and smooth skin. Instead of wasting dollars purchasing expensive creams and pills that claim to cure acne, adopt the paleo diet that will not only help get rid of the stubborn pimples but will also improve your overall health.

Clears Brain Fog

With our stressful and busy lifestyles, we once in a while experience brain fog – a condition that makes you forgetful. This is usually caused by lack of proper nourishment to your brain. You now see that every part of your body, however small or big it might be, requires you to provide it with healthy meals that are loaded with essential nutrients.

Paleo diet is packed with essential nutrients and that's exactly what you literally need to jumpstart your brain!

As for how the paleo diet/approach is beneficial to our health, I could go on and on, but I want you to embrace it and discover on your own other benefits of the approach!

14 Day Paleo Diet Meal Plan

This is the never before revealed Paleo Diet Plan. You will get rapid results since the diet exclude refined , processed foods, sugar, legumes, grains ,unhealthy flours and oils.

You need to start your Breakfast healthy with Herbal tea .Then fill up your Breakfast with Smoothies /Omelet /vegie or fruit bowls. Lunches and Diets consist with Veggies, Fish or Meat. So if you stick to the plan you will shed your pounds. On top of that if you do regular exercise you will see rapid results even sooner. Paleo life style encourages you to have exercises so that it motivate and point you at the right direction to reach your fitness goals while staying true to the diet.

 It is recommended that you drink at least 8 glasses of water per day and have lots of fruits and veggies in between meals as snacks to reduce Weight.

It's important to determine the amount of pounds you need to shed. Write down your goal. Visualize yourself with the perfect weight while you stick to the diet plan. I strongly suggest if you decide to start your diet plan today mark it in your calendar and determine that you are going to stick to the 14 days and decide when you will be completing the diet and mark it in your calendar and discipline yourself. Once you make up your mind you are half way through since you will not allow yourself to eat unhealthy food even if someone offers to you. If you want to be Paleo food lover you need to avoid all the unhealthy Paleo food I have mentioned from now on. So that you know you have to follow the process during these 14 days. Stick to the pan and you will eventually get there even without your knowledge.

I hope you will achieve your desired goal of losing weight and enjoy this delicious and healthy diet plan.

14 Day Paleo Diet Meal Plan

(Best viewed in landscape mode)

DAY	BREAKFAST	AM SNACK/ DETOX DRINK	LUNCH	PM SNACK/ DETOX DRINK	DINNER	BEDTIME SNACK/DET OX DRINK
DAY 1	1 Cup Paleo Herbal Tea 1 Serving Delicious Paleo Zucchini Smoothie	Sesame Crackers 1 glass (250ml) coconut water	1 Serving Kale, Cranberr y, and Sweet Potato Salad 2 Glass of Water	1 glass (250ml) Paleo Almond Milk	2 Sesame Salmon Burgers	1 serving Pickled Veggies
DAY 2	1 Cup Paleo Herbal Tea 1 Serving Avocado Shrimp Omelet 1 Serving Healthy Paleo Green Smoothie	1 glass (250ml) Paleo Raw Mango Lassie	1 serving Mustard Crusted Salmon with Arugula and Spinach Salad 2 Glass Water	1 serving Stuffed Celery Bites	Spiced Chicken w/ Grilled Lime 2 Glass Water	1 glass (250ml) Mango Lassie
DAY 3	1 Cup Paleo Herbal Tea 1 serving Healthy Paleo Tropical Smoothie	A handful of mixed berries (blueberries ,raspberries, blackberries ,strawberries)	1 bowl Butternu t Squash Soup 1 serving Tomato & Tuna Burgers 2 Glass Water	1 glass (250ml) Matcha Pineapple Mango Smoothie	1 serving Asian Stir Fry 2 Glass Water	1 serving Healthy Spiced Nuts

DAY 4	1 Cup Paleo Herbal Tea Ultimate Quinoa Veggie Breakfast Bowl	1 glass (250ml) Paleo Strawberry Clementine Smoothie	1 Serving Shawarma Chicken w/ Lemon-Basil Vinaigrette 2 Glass Water	1 serving Pesto-Stuffed Mushrooms	1 serving Turkey Hash 2 Glass Water	1 Serving Healthy Fried Plantain
DAY 5	1 Cup Paleo Herbal Tea 1 Serving Thick and Creamy Strawberry Chia Banana Smoothie	1 serving Healthy Sautéed Kale	1 bowl Roasted Broccoli w/ Lemon 2 Glass Water	A handful of mixed berries (blueberries ,raspberries, blackberries ,strawberries)	1 serving Fried Chili Beef w/ Cashews 2 Glass Water	1 serving Guacamole w/ Vegetables
DAY 6	1 Cup Paleo Herbal Tea 1 serving Paleo Strawberry Clementine Smoothie Glass	1 (250ml) Hydration Juice	1 Serving Chicken & Broccoli 2 Glass Water	Handful Brazil nuts 1 apple sprinkled with cinnamon	1 Serving Turkey Lettuce Wraps 2 Glass Water	1 Serving Fig Tapenade
DAY 7	1 Cup Paleo Herbal Tea 1 Serving Avocado Shrimp Omelet	1 serving Curried Roasted Cauliflower	1 Serving Salmon w/ Chanterelle Mushrooms 2 Glass Water	1 glass (250ml) Berry Delicious	1 Serving Asian Mince Curry 2 Glass Water	1 serving Veggie Snack

DAY 8	1 Cup Paleo Herbal Tea 1 glass (250ml) Paleo Rainbow Smoothie	1 glass (250ml) Orange Juice	1 Serving Hamburger Veggie Casserole 2 Glass Water	1 glass (250ml) freshly squeezed lemon juice	1 serving Gingery Chicken & Veggies 2 Glass Water	1 glass (250ml) Berry Delicious
DAY 9	1 Cup Paleo Herbal Tea 1 Serve Paleo Pumpkin Smoothie	1 serving Squash Fries	1 Serving Red Snapper in Sauce 2 Glass Water	1 glass (250ml) Blueberry Coconut Milk Smoothie	1 Serving Fish with Herb sauce 2 Glass Water	1 serving Fig Tapenade
DAY 10	1 Cup Paleo Herbal Tea 1 Glass Berry Delicious Smoothie	1 glass (250ml) Date Orange Smoothie	1 serving Grilled Lemony Chicken 2 Glass Water	1 serving Roasted Asparagus	1 serving Asian Stir Fry 2 Glass Water	1 glass (250ml) Paleo Strawberry Lemonade
DAY 11	1 Cup Paleo Herbal Tea 1 Serving Turkey Scrambled Egg	1 serving Roasted Balsamic Beets	1 Serving Roasted Seafood w/ Herbs &Lemon 2 Glass Water	1 Serving Paprika and chili kale chips	1 serving Ground Beef & Zucchini 2 Glass Water	1 serving sesame crackers
DAY 12	1 Cup Paleo Herbal Tea 1 Serving Paleo Strawberry Clementine Smoothie	1 Serving Baked Cinnamon Apple Chips	1 serving Avocado Chicken Salad 2 Glass Water	1serving Guacamole w/ Vegetables	1 serving Coconut-Crusted Cod 2 Glass Water	1 glass (250ml) Freshly Squeezed orange juice

DAY 13	1 Cup Paleo Herbal Tea 1 Serving The Best Western Omelet. 1 glass Paleo Green Juice	1 Serving Roasted Asparagus	1 bowl Cucumber & Avocado Salad 2 Glass Water	1 glass (250ml) Paleo Tropical Smoothie	1 serving Curried Chicken Salad 2 Glass Water	1 serving Vinegar & Salt Kale Chips
DAY 14	1 Cup Paleo Herbal Tea 1 Serving Healthy Paleo Green Smoothie	1 Serving Chicken Liver Pâté	1 serving Coconut Chicken w/ Mustard-Honey Sauce 2 Glass Water	1 serving Roasted Sweet Potato Chips	1 serving Mexican Chicken Served With 'Rice' 2 Glass Water	1 glass (250ml) Freshly Squeezed Lemon Juice

PALEO DIET BREAKFAST RECIPES

Palo Delicious Zucchini Smoothie

Yields: 2 Servings

Prep Time: 5 Minutes

Ingredients:

- 1 Large Zucchini
- 1 Brown Onion
- 2 Tbs Coconut Oil
- 2 Cups of water

Directions

Rinse and pat dry and cut the Zucchini into slices. Chop the onion. Heat the coconut oil in a pan under moderate heat and fry the onions until golden brown. Add the Zucchini and cook under medium heat until tender. Add 2 cups of water and boil. When boiling blend together .Add a dash of salt to taste. Enjoy!

Paleo Rainbow Smoothie

Yields: 4 Servings

Prep Time: 5 Minutes

Ingredients:

- 1/2 cup almond milk
- 2 cups fresh spinach
- 1 fresh banana
- 1 cup fresh blackberries
- 1 cup fresh strawberries

Directions

Rinse and pat dry the berries and spinach.

To create different colored layers: start by blending together a splash of almond milk and strawberries; pour into serving glasses.

Next, blend together a splash of almond milk and blackberries; pour onto the strawberry mixture.

Finally, blend together spinach, bananas, and the remaining almond milk; pour onto the blackberries.

Garnish each glass with a strawberry and enjoy!

Healthy Paleo Green Smoothie

Yields: 2 Servings

Prep Time: 20 Minutes

Ingredients

- 1/2 mango
- 1 kiwi fruit
- 1/2 banana
- ¼ tin pineapple (500g)
- 2 red apples
- 1/2 bunches kale
- Handful spinach
- 1 carrot
- 1/2 pear
- 1/2 peach
- 1/4 papaya

Directions

Rinse the fruit and cut into juicer-sized pieces.

Run all the ingredients through a juicer; stir together in a pitcher.

Refrigerate the juice for at least 2 hours before serving.

Paleo Tropical Smoothie

Yields: 2 glasses

Prep Time: 10 Minutes

Ingredients

- 2 cups water
- Juice of 1 small lemon
- 2 large kale leaves
- 2 tbsp. flax seeds
- 1/2 tsp. freshly grated ginger
- 1 pear
- 1 apple

Directions

Cut pear and apple into four equal parts; remove seeds and stems and add to the blender or food processor.

Add all the remaining ingredients and process until very smooth. Add extra water if necessary.

For taste variations, add other fresh fruit, fresh herbs, coconut, slivered almonds or any dark leafy greens.

Matcha Pineapple Mango Smoothie

Yields: 2 glasses

Ingredients

- 1/2 to 1 cup water
- 1 cup pineapple
- 1 tbsp. pineapple juice
- 1 cup frozen mango chunks
- 1 tsp. honey
- 1 tbsp. protein powder (Optional)
- 1.25 tsp. matcha green tea

Directions

Chop up all the fresh fruit and blend all together in a blender. Enjoy!

Avocado Shrimp Omelet

Yields: 2 Servings

Total Time: 40 Minutes

Prep Time: 10 Minutes

Cook Time: 30 Minutes

Ingredients

*   1/4 pound shrimp, peeled and de-veined
*   2 large free range eggs, beaten
*   1/2 medium avocado, diced
*   1 medium   tomato, diced
*   1 tsp. coconut oil
*   1/8 tsp. freshly ground black pepper
*   1/4 tsp. sea salt
*   1 tbsp. Freshly chopped cilantro

Directions

Cook shrimp in a skillet set over medium heat until it turns pink; chop the cooked shrimp and set aside.

In a small bowl, toss together avocado, tomato, and cilantro; season with sea salt and pepper and set aside.

In a separate bowl, beat the eggs and set aside.

Set a skillet over medium heat; add coconut oil and heat until hot.

Add half of the egg to the skillet and tilt the skillet to cover the bottom. When almost cooked, add shrimp onto one side of the egg and fold in half. Cook for 1 minute more and top with the avocado-tomato mixture.

Repeat with the remaining ingredients for the second omelet. Serve with prepared Avocado, tomato and Cilantro.

Paleo Almond and Banana Smoothie

Yields: 1 Serving

Prep Time: 5 Minutes

Ingredients

- ½ cup unsweetened almond milk
- 2 tbsp. pumpkin puree
- 1 tsp. honey
- 1 frozen banana
- ½ tsp. vanilla extract
- ¼ tsp. nutmeg
- ¼ tsp. cloves
- ¼ tsp. cinnamon
- 1 tbsp. hemp hearts

Directions

Combine together all ingredients in a food processor or blender and pulse until very smooth.

Pour the smoothie into a tall serving glass and enjoy!

Paleo Strawberry Clementine Smoothie

Yields: 1 Serving

Prep Time: 5 Minutes

Ingredients

- 8 oz. strawberries – frozen or fresh

- 1 banana, frozen, chopped into chunks

- 2 Clementine's or Mandarins

Directions

Thaw the frozen banana chunks for at least 5 minutes. Slightly defrost the frozen strawberries.

In the meantime, peel clementine's and remove seeds.

Combine together all the ingredients in a blender and pulse until very smooth.

Pineapple and Coconut milk Smoothie

Yields: 2 servings

Prep Time: 5 Minutes

Ingredients

*   3/4 cup pineapple, frozen

*   3/4 cup coconut milk

Directions

Combine together all ingredients in a blender and blend on high speed until very smooth. Pour the smoothie into a tall serving glass and serve.

Healthy Paleo Smoothie

Yields: 2 Servings

Prep Time: 5 Minutes

Ingredients

- 1 banana

- 1 cup coconut water

- Juice of 1 lime

- 1 peeled and quartered orange

- 1 1/2 cups frozen or fresh pineapple chunks

- ½ tsp. nutmeg

- 1 tbsp. ginger

- 4 ice cubes

Directions

Blend together all ingredients in a blender until very smooth. Add a little more water to attain the desired consistency. Divide between two serving glasses and enjoy.

Berry Delicious Smoothie

Yields: 2 cups

Prep Time: 5 Minutes

Ingredients

- 200ml coconut Water
- Drop vanilla essence
- Handful ice
- Handful mixed frozen berries

Directions

Blend together all ingredients in a blender until very smooth. Add a little coconut milk if you like the smoothie to be thick. Enjoy!

Blueberry and Coconut Water Smoothie

Yields: 2 Servings

Total Time: 5 Minutes

Prep Time: 5 Minutes

Ingredients

- 2 bananas

- 1 14 oz. can coconut water

- 1 cup frozen blueberries

- 14 ice cubes

Directions

Blend together all ingredients in a blender until very smooth. Enjoy!

Avocado and Almond Omelet

Yields: 2 Servings

Total Time: 12 Minutes

Prep Time: 2 Minutes

Cook Time: 10 Minutes

Ingredients

- 3 large free range eggs
- 1/2 medium avocado, sliced
- 1/2 cup sliced almonds
- Salt and Pepper

Directions

Set a nonstick skillet over medium high heat.

In a bowl, beat the eggs and pour into the skillet; cook for about 1 minute and reduce heat to medium low; cook for 4 minutes more.

Top with avocado and almonds. Serve sprinkled with sea salt and freshly ground pepper.

Quinoa Veggie Breakfast Bowl

Yields: 1 serving

Ingredients

- 1/2 cup quinoa, rinsed

- 1/2 cup water

- 1/2 cup Coconut milk

- 1 egg

- ½ cup sliced mushrooms

- ¼ cup broccoli, chopped

- Salt & pepper

Directions

Add olive oil to a skillet set over medium heat. Add mushrooms and broccoli and stir-fry for about 5 minutes or until cooked through. Remove the skillet from heat and set aside.

In a saucepan, combine quinoa, water and coconut milk; bring to a gentle boil and lower heat to low. Simmer until almost all liquid is absorbed.

Stir in veggies, cheese, and salt and pepper until well combined. Cover and set aside.

Fry the egg sunny-side up.

Serve quinoa in a bowl topped with the egg.

Blueberry & Dates- Breakfast cereal

Yields: 4 Servings

Total Time: 50 Minutes

Prep Time: 20 Minutes

Cook Time: 30 Minutes

Ingredients

- 1/2 cup dried blueberries
- 1/2 cup unsweetened coconut flakes
- 1 cup   pumpkin seeds
- 2 cups almond flour
- 6 medium dates, pitted
- 1/3 cup coconut oil
- 2 tsp. Cinnamon
- 1 tbsp. vanilla
- 1/2 tsp. sea salt

Directions

Preheat your oven to 325°F.

Add coconut oil, dates and half the almond flour to a food processor and mix it thoroughly. Add pumpkin seeds and continue pulsing until roughly chopped.

Transfer the mixture to a large bowl and add cinnamon, vanilla and salt; spread on a baking sheet and bake for about 20m minutes or until browned. Remove from the oven and let cool slightly before stirring in blueberries and coconut.

Ultimate Paleo Almond Flour Muffins

Yield: 10 Muffins

Total Time: 23 Minutes

Prep Time: 5 Minutes

Cook Time: 18 Minutes

Ingredients

• 2-1/2 cups almond meal or flour

• ⅓ cup unsweetened pumpkin puree

• 3 large free-range eggs

• 2 tbsp. Melted coconut oil

• 1 tsp. apple cider vinegar

• 2 tbsp. honey or maple syrup

• ½ tsp. sea salt

• ¾ tsp. baking soda

• Optional Stir-Ins: 1 cup fresh fruit (diced apple or blueberries)

• Optional Flavorings: citrus zest, 1 tsp. almond or vanilla extract, spice (cumin or cinnamon), or dried herbs (such as dill, basil)

Direction:

Preheat your oven to 350°F. Prepare 10 muffin cups in a standard 12-cup muffin tin by lining then with paper liners.

Whisk together almond flour, salt and baking soda (and any dried spices or herbs, if using).

Wisk together eggs, vinegar, extra virgin olive oil, honey, and pumpkin in a small bowl (whisk in any zest or extracts at this point, if using).

Stir the wet ingredients into the dry mixture until well blended.

Divide the batter among the prepared cups and bake for about 18 minutes or until the edges are golden brown and the centers set.

Transfer the tin to a cooling rack and let the muffins cool for at least 30 minutes before removing.

Turkey Scrambled Eggs

Yields: 2 Servings

Total Time: 30 Minutes

Prep Time: 15 Minutes

Cook Time: 15 Minutes

Ingredients

- 1 tbsp. coconut oil
- 200g pound minced turkey,
- 1 medium red bell pepper, diced
- 1/2 medium yellow onion, diced
- 1/4 tsp. hot pepper sauce
- 3 large free range eggs
- 1/4 tsp. black pepper, freshly ground
- 1/4 tsp. sea salt

Directions

Set a medium pan over medium high heat; add coconut oil and sauté onions until fragrant.

Add turkey and red pepper; cook until turkey is done.

In the meantime, beat eggs in a bowl; stir in salt and pepper.

Pour the eggs into the pan with turkey, peppers, and onions. Gently scramble the eggs until cooked.

To serve, top with hot sauce.

Tapioca Crêpes

Yields: 2 Servings

Total Time: 35 Minutes

Prep Time: 10 Minutes

Cook Time: 25 Minutes

Ingredients

- 1 large free range egg

- 1 cup full fat coconut milk

- 1 cup tapioca flour

- 1/4 tsp. sea salt

- Toppings of choice- for crepes, (I prefer almond butter and berries, but you can also mix it up with cinnamon, applesauce, sautéed veggies, etc.)

Directions

In a medium bowl, mix together all the ingredients.

Set a skillet over medium heat and add 1/3 cup of the mixture when hot, tilting the skillet to spread out the batter.

Cook both sides for about 4 minutes or until lightly browned.

Serve warm topped with desired ingredients.

Thick & Creamy Strawberry Banana Shake

Yield: 1 to 2 Servings

Total Time: 5 Minutes

Prep Time: 5 Minutes

Cook Time: 0 Minutes

Ingredients

- ½ tbsp. ground chia seeds
- ½ tsp. vanilla extract
- 1 scoop vanilla protein powder (Optional)
- ½ cup orange juice
- 1 banana, frozen
- ⅔ cup almond milk
- ½ cup frozen strawberries

Directions

Combine all ingredients in a blender and blend until very smooth. Enjoy!

Pumpkin and Banana Smoothie

Yields: 2 Servings

Total Time: 5 Minutes

Prep Time: 5 Minutes

Cook Time: 0 Minutes

Ingredients

- 1 tbsp. honey or maple syrup
- 1 cup almond milk
- ⅓ cup pumpkin puree
- 1 frozen banana
- 1 heaping scoop vanilla protein powder (Optional)

Directions

Combine all ingredients in a blender and blend until very smooth. Enjoy!

Fennel Pork Apple Breakfast Patties

Yields: 8 2-inch patties

Total Time: 35 Minutes

Prep Time: 10 Minutes

Cook Time: 25 Minutes

Ingredients

- ½ red apple, diced

- 2 tsp. Fennel seeds

- 3 tbsp. coconut oil

- 2 tbsp. Maple syrup

- 450g ground pork (You can use Minced Chicken or Lamb if desired)

- 1 tsp. onion powder

- 1 tsp. garlic powder

- 1 tsp. paprika

- ½ tsp. dried rosemary

- ½ tsp. red pepper flakes

- ½ tsp. ground sage

- ¼ tsp. black pepper

- 1 tsp. sea salt

Directions

Toast fennel seeds in a sauté pan set over medium for about 5 minutes or until fragrant.

In a large bowl, combine all ingredient except coconut oil; flatten the mixture between your hands to make patties.

Melt coconut oil in a large skillet set over low heat; add three or four patties and cook about 6 minutes per side or until cooked through and golden brown.

The Best Western Omelet

Yields: 2 Servings

Total Time: 35 Minutes

Prep Time: 10 Minutes

Cook Time: 25 Minutes

Ingredients

- 1/4 pound cooked and diced turkey/chicken
- 1 cup chopped spinach
- 1 medium tomato, diced
- 1 medium bell pepper, diced
- 1/2 medium yellow onion, diced
- 3 large free range eggs
- 1 tsp. Coconut oil
- 1/4 tsp. freshly ground black pepper
- 1/4 tsp. sea salt

Directions

Rinse and chop the vegetables; set aside.

In a small bowl beat the eggs until well blended; set aside.

Set a skillet over medium heat; heat the coconut oil.

Add half of the eggs to the pan and tilt to cover the bottom of the pan. When almost set, add half of the chicken/turkey and vegetables to one side of the omelet and cook until the egg is set. Fold the empty side over the top of the veggies and ham and cook for 2 minutes longer.

Repeat with the remaining ingredients and serve warm.

Blueberries & Raspberries pancakes

Ingredients

* ¼ cup blueberries

* ¼ cup raspberries

* ½ tbsp. chopped almonds

* ½ cup almond milk

* 250g almond flour

* 2 egg whites

* 1 Tbs Coconut Oil

* ½ tsp Salt

Directions

Mix the milk and almond flour together, stir in the egg whites and salt .Add the berries and chopped almonds. Melt coconut oil in a large skillet set over low heat .Make pan cakes. Enjoy!

Chocolate Chia Cherry Shake

Yields: 2 Shakes

Total Time: 5 Minutes

Prep Time: 5 Minutes

Cook Time: 0 Minutes

Ingredients

- 1 tbsp. Ground chia seeds
- 1 tsp. unsweetened cocoa powder
- 1½ cup almond milk
- 1 cup pitted cherries, frozen
- 1 tbsp. honey, to sweeten
- 1 scoop chocolate protein powder (Optional)

Directions

Combine all the ingredients in a blender and blend until very smooth. Enjoy!

Honey and Chia smoothie topping with Fruit and Nut

Ingredients

- 1/2 tbsp. honey
- 1 cup coconut milk
- 1/4 cup chia seeds
- Any Fruit
- 1 tsp chopped Nuts

Directions

In a bowl, combine together honey, coconut milk and chia seeds; refrigerate overnight. To serve, top with nuts and fruit.

Easy Chicken Breakfast Casserole

Yields: 2 to 3 Servings

Total Time: 50 Minutes

Prep Time: 25 Minutes

Cook Time: 25 Minutes

Ingredients

- 250g Ground Chicken
- 1 Medium yam or sweet potato, diced
- 1 tbsp. melted coconut oil
- 4 eggs, whisked
- ½ tsp. garlic powder
- 1 cups chopped spinach
- ½ yellow onion, diced
- ½ tsp. Sea salt

Directions

Preheat your oven to 400°F. Coat a 9x12 baking dish with Olive oil.

Toss the diced sweet potatoes in coconut oil and sprinkle with salt; transfer to the baking sheet and bake for about 25 minutes or until tender.

In the meantime, set a sauté pan over medium heat; add yellow onion and sauté for about 4 minutes or until fragrant. Stir in minced chicken and cook for about 5 minutes or until the chicken is no longer pink.

Transfer the chicken mixture to the baking dish and add spinach and sweet potatoes. Top with eggs and sprinkle with garlic powder and salt. Mix until well combined and bake for about 30 minutes or until the eggs are set in the center.

Tomato Dill Frittata

Yields: 2 Servings

Total Time: 45 Minutes

Prep Time: 10 Minutes

Cook Time: 35 Minutes

Ingredients

- 2 tbsp. chopped fresh chives

- 2 tbsp. chopped fresh dill

- 2 tomatoes, diced

- 4 free-range eggs, whisked

- 1 tsp. red pepper flakes

- 2 garlic cloves, minced

- 1/4 cup crumbled goat cheese, optional

- Coconut oil, for greasing the pan

- Sea salt

- Black pepper

Directions

Preheat your oven to 325°F. Grease a cast iron skillet or saucepan and set aside.

In a large bowl, whisk together the eggs; beat in the remaining ingredients until well mixed.

Pour the egg mixture into the prepared pan and bake for about 35 minutes or until cooked through. Garnish the frittata with extra chives and dill to serve.

Chicken, Leek and Asparagus Dill Breakfast Casserole

Yields: 2 to 3 Servings

Total Time: 50 Minutes

Prep Time: 10 Minutes

Cook Time: 40 Minutes

Ingredients

*   Coconut oil, for greasing the dish

*   250g Minced Chicken

*   ¼ cup coconut milk

*   4 free range eggs, beaten

*   1 tbsp. minced fresh dill

*   3-4 stalks asparagus, chopped

*   1 thinly sliced leek

*   ¼ tsp. garlic powder

*   Sea salt and pepper

Directions

Preheat your oven to 325°F. Grease a square baking dish and set aside.

Place the chicken mince in a pan set over medium heat; break them into small pieces. Cook for a few minutes and add asparagus and leeks; continue cooking for about 5 minutes more or until chicken is no longer pink. Remove the pan from heat, discarding excess fat.

Whisk together eggs, garlic powder, dill, coconut milk, salt and pepper in a bowl; pour the mixture into the prepared baking dish and add the chicken mixture; mix well and bake for about 40 minutes or until set in the center.

Zucchini Frittata

Yield: 9x13 inch pizza frittata (2-4 Servings)

Total Time: 55 Minutes

Prep Time: 10 Minutes

Cook Time: 45 Minutes

Ingredients

- 2 medium (about 2 pounds sliced) zucchini
- 4 crushed garlic cloves
- 2 cups tomato puree
- 4 free range eggs
- 2 tbsp. extra virgin olive oil
- 3 tbsp. freshly chopped oregano
- 1/2 cup chopped basil
- 2 tsp. sea salt
- Optional: Nutritional yeast

Directions

Preheat your oven to 350°F.

In a bowl, beat the eggs; whisk in tomato puree along with the remaining ingredients except zucchini.

Pour about one third of the egg mixture into a 9x13 inch pan and spread until the bottom is covered.

Line the baking pan with zucchini slices and wiggle to settle the zucchini into the mixture. Add another one third of the egg mixture, and cover with another layer of zucchini. Top with remaining egg mixture and bake for about 45 minutes or until cooked through.

Remove the frittata from the oven and cut into squares to serve.

Leek & Arugula Frittata

Yields: 2 Servings

Total Time: 45 Minutes

Prep Time: 10 Minutes

Cook Time: 35 Minutes

Ingredients

- 1 tsp. Balsamic vinegar
- 2 tbsp. extra virgin olive oil
- 2 tbsp. coconut oil
- 1/2 cup full fat coconut milk
- 1/2 cup halved grape or cherry tomatoes
- 4 large free range eggs
- 2 cups chopped baby arugula
- 2 medium garlic cloves, minced
- ½ cup chopped medium leek
- 1/8 tsp. sea salt
- 1/8 tsp. black pepper

Directions

Preheat your oven to 350°F.

In a bowl, beat together the eggs, coconut milk and sea salt until well blended.

Melt coconut oil in a skillet set over medium heat; add leeks and sauté until tender. Add garlic and continue sautéing for about 1 minute or until fragrant. Add the egg mixture and sprinkle with sea salt and pepper.

Transfer the pan to the oven and bake for about 25 minutes or until the eggs are set.

Remove from oven and let stand for at least 5 minutes. Top with chopped tomatoes and arugula.

In a bowl, whisk together extra virgin olive oil and vinegar; drizzle over the frittata and serve.

Broccoli & Chicken Quiche

Serves: 4 slices

Ingredients

- 2 tbsp. coconut oil
- 1 cups almond flour
- 1/2 cup broccoli
- 3 free range eggs
- 350g minced chicken
- 2 tbsp. water
- 1 tsp. sea salt

Directions

Cook the chicken and set aside.

Steam the broccoli and set aside.

Blend almond flour and sea salt in a food processor until well combined.

Add one egg and coconut oil and continue processing to form a ball.

Spread the dough on a quiche dish and top with broccoli and chicken mince.

In a bowl, whisk the remaining eggs with water and pour over the broccoli and chicken mince.

Bake at 350°Ffor about 35 minutes or until firm and cooked through.

PALEO LUNCH RECIPES

Beef and Veggie Casserole

Yields: 2 Servings

Total Time: 30 Minutes

Prep Time: 10 Minutes

Cook Time: 20 Minutes

Ingredients

- 1 lb. ground beef
- 1 tbsp. extra virgin olive oil
- 3 tbsp. minced garlic
- 1/2 cup diced onions
- 1 cup sliced purple cabbage
- 1 chopped red pepper
- 1/2 cup chopped fresh oregano
- Sea salt
- Freshly cracked black pepper

Directions

Preheat your oven 350°F.

Brown beef in a saucepan; strain off fat and set aside.

Meanwhile, chop oregano, garlic, onions, cabbage, and pepper in a large bowl; set aside.

Grease a 9×13 inch baking dish with extra virgin olive oil and layer vegetables and hamburger until all ingredients are used up.

Bake for about 20 minutes or until the vegetables are warmed but crunchy.

Garnish with some dried Italian herbs.

Roasted Broccoli w/ Lemon

Yields: 3 Servings

Total Time: 30 Minutes

Prep Time: 10 Minutes

Cook Time: 20 Minutes

Ingredients

- 2 Heads of broccoli, chopped into florets
- 2 tsp. freshly squeezed lemon juice
- 2 tsp. freshly grated lemon zest
- 4 minced cloves garlic
- 1/4 cup extra virgin olive oil
- A pinch of sea salt
- A pinch of freshly ground black pepper

Directions

Preheat your oven to 400°F.

Place broccoli onto a rimmed baking sheet and drizzle with extra virgin olive oil; sprinkle with lemon zest, garlic, sea salt and pepper and toss to coat well.

Bake for about 20 minutes, turning once, until broccoli florets are slightly browned.

Transfer the baked broccoli to a large bowl and toss with lemon juice. Serve warm.

Coconut Chicken w/ Mustard- Honey Sauce

Yields: 2 Servings

Total Time: 35 Minutes

Prep Time: 20 Minutes

Cook Time: 15 Minutes

Ingredients

•   2 boneless and skinless chicken breasts, sliced into small strips

•   1 cup unsweetened coconut flakes

•   2 free range eggs

•   1/2 cup coconut flour

•   1/2 cup Dijon mustard

•   1/2 cup honey

•   1 cup steamed vegetables for serving, optional

Directions

Preheat your oven to 400°F and line baking sheet with parchment paper.

Rinse the chicken and slice into small strips; pat them dry and set aside.

Place coconut flour onto a plate and set aside.

In a bowl, whisk the eggs and set aside.

Place coconut flakes in another plate and set aside.

Dip the chicken strips into the coconut flour, then into the eggs and finally into coconut flakes; arrange them onto the prepared baking sheet and bake for about 15 minutes or until browned.

Meanwhile, combine honey and mustard in a bowl; drizzle over the baked chicken strips and serve with steamed veggies.

Chicken and Broccoli

Yields: 2 Servings

Total Time: 35 Minutes

Prep Time: 15 Minutes

Cook Time: 20 Minutes

Ingredients

- 1 cup broccoli, cut into florets
- 1 pound chicken breasts cut into small strips
- Coconut oil
- A pinch of freshly ground black pepper
- 1 medium orange
- A pinch of sea salt
- 1/2 minced ginger
- 2 tbsp. apple cider vinegar

Directions

Add coconut to a skillet set over medium high heat; add the chicken and sauté for about 4 minutes.

Add broccoli, ginger, apple cider vinegar and orange juice. Season with salt and pepper and continue sautéing until the chicken is cooked through.

Kale, Cranberry, and Sweet Potato Salad

Yields: 6 Servings

Total Time: 20 Minutes

Prep Time: 20 Minutes

Cook Time: 0 Minutes

Ingredients

- 2 large peeled sweet potatoes, cubed
- 2 bunches kale, chopped into small pieces
- 1 tbsp. freshly squeezed lemon juice
- 3 tbsp. extra virgin olive oil
- 1/4 cup Sunflower seeds
- 1/2 cup dried cranberries
- 1 tsp. Dijon mustard
- A pinch of sea salt
- A pinch of freshly ground pepper

Directions

Place the potatoes in a medium saucepan and cover with water; stir in a pinch of salt and bring to a gentle boil. Lower heat to a simmer and simmer for about 15 minutes or until the potatoes are tender; drain and let cool.

In a large bowl, whisk together mustard, lemon juice and extra virgin olive oil.

Add the sweet potatoes along with all the remaining ingredients; toss to mix well and serve.

Mustard Crusted Salmon with Arugula and Spinach Salad

Yields: 1 Serving

Total Time: 45 Minutes

Prep Time: 15 Minutes

Cook Time: 20 Minutes

Ingredients

For Salmon

- 15 oz. salmon filet
- 1 tbsp. coarse ground mustard
- A pinch of sea salt

For Salad

- 2 tbsp. Dried cranberries
- 2 tbsp. chopped pecans
- 1/2 cup chopped baby spinach
- 1 cup chopped arugula

For Dressing

- 1 tbsp. extra virgin olive oil
- 1 tbsp. white wine vinegar
- 1 tbsp. Dijon mustard

Directions

Preheat your oven to 350°F.

Grease a baking sheet with extra virgin olive oil and place in salmon filet; pat dry with paper towels and sprinkle with ground mustard, covering the entire top if fish. Bake for about

15 minutes or until fish flakes easily with a fork.

Meanwhile, whisk together the dressing ingredients and set aside.

Combine together the salad ingredients in a mixing bowl; add in the dressing and toss until well coated. Spoon your salad onto a serving bowl and top with salmon. Enjoy! While the salmon is cooking, whisk together the ingredients for the dressing. Set aside.

Sautéed Kale

Yields: 2 Servings

Total Time: 30 Minutes

Prep Time: 15 Minutes

Cook Time: 15 Minutes

Ingredients

- 4 cups rinsed and chopped kale
- 2 tbsp. sliced almonds
- 1 tbsp. red wine vinegar
- 1 tbsp. extra virgin olive oil
- 2 garlic cloves, minced
- 1/4 onion, diced
- A pinch of sea salt to taste

Directions

Heat extra virgin olive oil in a medium skillet set over medium heat; add onion and sauté for about 5 minutes or until translucent.

Add kale, garlic, almonds and vinegar and cook for about 7 minutes or until kale is tender. Season with sea salt to serve.

Avocado Chicken Salad

Yields: 4 Servings

Total Time: 45 Minutes

Prep Time: 45 Minutes

Cook Time: 0 Minutes

Ingredients

- 4 boneless and skinless chicken thighs
- 3 medium avocados
- 1 tbsp. avocado oil
- 1/2 red onion, diced
- 2 small tomatoes, diced
- 1 tsp. chili powder
- 1 tsp. cumin
- Freshly squeezed lime juice from 1 lime
- A pinch of freshly ground black pepper
- A pinch of sea salt

Directions

Preheat your oven to 350°F.

Arrange chicken thighs in a baking dish and sprinkle with cumin, chili powder and sea salt. Drizzle with extra virgin olive oil and bake for about 30 minutes or until the chicken is cooked through.

Remove from oven and shred the chicken with two forks; set aside to cool.

Mash avocado in a bowl until smooth and creamy. Stir in lime juice, onion and tomato until well combined.

Remove from oven and shred the chicken with two forks; set aside to cool.

Mash avocado in a bowl until smooth and creamy. Stir in lime juice, onion and tomato until well combined. Add the chicken and stir well.

Season with salt and pepper and serve immediately.

Paleo Chinese Chicken Salad

Yields: 4 Servings

Total Time: 20 Minutes

Prep Time: 20 Minutes

Cook Time: 6 Minutes

Ingredients

- 1 rotisserie chicken, torn into shreds
- ½ cup cashews
- 2 tbsp. white sesame seeds
- 2 tbsp. black sesame seeds
- ½ cup chopped cilantro
- 1 head of Napa cabbage, thinly chopped
- 2 bags shredded carrots
- 5 chopped green onions, green, and white parts
- 1 tsp. Sirach
- 1 tsp. spicy chili oil
- 1 tbsp. toasted sesame oil
- 2 tbsp. hoisin sauce
- 3 tbsp. extra virgin olive oil
- 3 tbsp. finely minced ginger
- ¼ cup white wine vinegar
- ¼ cup tamari or regular soy sauce
- ½ tsp. sea salt

Directions

Make the dress: In a mason jar with a lid, mix extra virgin olive oil, minced garlic, vinegar, tamari, Sirach, hoisin sauce, chili oil, toasted sesame oil, chopped green onions and sea salt. Secure the lid and shake to mix well; set aside.

In a large plastic bag, combine shredded chicken, sesame seeds, shredded carrots, chopped cabbage, cashews, cilantro, and enough dressing; shake well to mix.

Serve the salad into bowls and enjoy!

Seared Tuna Nicosia Salad

Yields: 2 Servings

Total Time: 31 Minutes

Prep Time: 25 Minutes

Cook Time: 6 Minutes

Ingredients

- 2 cups petite lettuce leaves
- 2 ounces trimmed French green beans
- 2 tsp. capers
- 1 tbsp. extra-virgin olive oil
- 1/2 garlic clove, minced
- 1/4 tsp. maple syrup
- 1 tsp. Dijon mustard
- 1 tbsp. fresh lemon juice
- 8-ounce tuna steak
- 2 hard-boiled eggs, sliced
- 4 radishes, sliced thin
- 2 small cucumbers, thinly sliced crosswise
- 1/4 red onion, thinly sliced
- 1/2 cup cherry tomatoes, halved
- 1/4 cup fresh basil leaves
- Olive oil cooking spray
- Fresh cracked black pepper
- 1/4 tsp. sea salt

- 1 tsp. water

Direction

Bring a pot of water to a gentle boil; add beans and boil for about 2 minutes or until crisp-tender and bright green. Drain the beans and plunge into iced water; drain and set aside.

Arrange the lettuce, cucumbers, onion, tomatoes, basil, green beans, eggs, and radishes evenly between two serving plates.

Set a skillet over medium high heat and coat with olive oil cooking spray. Season tuna with sea salt and pepper and add to the pan; cook for about 2 minutes per side or until browned.

Cut cooked tuna across the grain and arrange over veggies.

Make the dressing: mix together lemon juice with other dressing ingredients in a jar and secure the lid; shake until well blended.

Drizzle the dressing over the salad and serve.

Tomato & Tuna Burgers

Yields: 6 Burgers

Total Time: 55 Minutes

Prep Time: 15 Minutes

Cook Time: 40 Minutes

Ingredients

- 1 tbsp. coconut flour
- 1 cup tuna, drained, rinsed
- 2 tbsp. Tomato paste
- 1 egg
- 1 garlic clove, crushed
- 1 small finely chopped red chili
- 1 small finely chopped red onion
- A pinch of freshly ground black pepper
- A pinch of sea salt

Optional for serving

- Extra chili
- Fresh coriander (cilantro)
- Avocado
- Lettuce

Direction

Preheat your oven to 350°F.Line a baking tray with parchment paper; set aside.

Combine burger ingredients in a bowl and stir to mix well.

Carefully roll and flatten tuna mixture with your hands into six, equal sized patties and arrange them on the mined baking tray. Bake for about 10 minutes or until cooked through.

To serve, place each burger into a lettuce leaf and top with sliced avocado, and sprinkle with extra slices of chili and fresh coriander.

Butternut Squash Soup

Yields: 6 Servings

Total Time: 55 Minutes

Prep Time: 15 Minutes

Cook Time: 40 Minutes

Ingredients

•   1 can (14-ounce) light coconut milk

•   3 pounds butternut squash, peeled, seeded, and sliced into small chunks

•   1 cup low-sodium vegetable broth

•   1 cup low-sodium chicken broth

•   3 cloves garlic, minced

•   2 tsp. Extra virgin olive oil

•   1 cup sliced shallots

•   1/2 tsp. sea salt

•   1 bay leaf

Optional garnishes:

•   Sunflower seeds

•   Fresh ground black pepper

•   Paprika

•   Cilantro

Direction

Preheat your oven to 450°F.

In a rimmed baking sheet, toss together onion, squash, 1 teaspoon oil and salt. Roast for about 30 minutes or until tender and browned.

Transfer the roasted veggies to a saucepan and add the remaining oil; cook over medium low heat, stirring regularly for about 5 minutes. Stir in garlic and cook for about 30 seconds. Stir in coconut milk, broths and bay leaf; cook for about 2 minutes; lower heat and simmer for about 5 minutes more. Discard bay leaf and transfer the mixture to a blender; blend until very smooth. Enjoy.

Shawarma Chicken with Lemon- Basil Vinaigrette

Yields: 4 Servings

Total Time: 45 Minutes

Prep Time: 35 Minutes

Cook Time: 10 Minutes

Ingredients

Chicken shawarma

- 2 tbsp. extra virgin olive oil
- 1 lb. free-range chicken breast, sliced into small strips
- 3 garlic cloves, minced
- 2 tbsp. freshly squeezed lemon juice
- ¼ tsp. ground coriander
- ½ tsp. ground cumin
- 1 tsp. curry powder
- ¾ tsp. sea salt

Salad

- 1 medium avocado, sliced
- 2 handfuls roughly torn fresh basil leaves
- 1 cup halved cherry tomatoes
- 6 cups spring greens

Lemon- Basil Vinaigrette

- 1 clove garlic, smashed
- 2 handfuls fresh basil leaves
- 5 tbsp. extra virgin olive oil

- 2 tbsp. freshly squeezed lemon juice
- ½ tsp. sea salt

Directions

Whisk together lemon juice, extra virgin olive oil, coriander, cumin, curry powder, garlic and sea salt in a bowl until well combined.

Combine the marinade with chicken strips in a sealable container; refrigerate, covered, for at least 20 minutes.

When ready, heat a skillet over medium high heat and add a small amount of extra virgin olive oil; add the chicken and cook, turning regularly, for about 8 minutes or until juices run clear.

Meanwhile, make the vinaigrette: in a blender or food processor, blend lemon juice, garlic, basil, and salt until smooth. Slowly add the oil and continue blending until well combined; set aside.

Make the salad: in a serving bowl, toss the greens with salt and pepper; top with chicken, avocado, tomatoes and basil.

Drizzle with the lemon-basil vinaigrette and enjoy!

Red Snapper in Sauce

Yields: 4 Servings

Total Time: 35 Minutes

Prep Time: 15 Minutes

Cook Time: 20 Minutes

Ingredients

• 2 lb. red snapper filets

• ¼ cup canola or extra virgin olive oil

• ½ red bell pepper, chopped

• ½ green bell pepper, chopped

• 4 scallions, thinly sliced

• 2 tomatoes, diced

• 2 cloves garlic

• 2 tbsp. freshly squeezed lemon juice

• ½ cup freshly squeezed lime juice

• 1 tsp. cayenne pepper

• 1 tsp. freshly ground black pepper

• Cilantro for garnish

Directions

Add extra virgin olive oil to a skillet and sauté garlic for about 4 minutes or until golden brown. Place fish in the oil and drizzle with lemon and lime juice. Sprinkle with black pepper and cayenne pepper and top with green and red bell peppers, scallions, and tomatoes.

Cover the skillet and simmer for about 15 minutes or until the fish flakes easily with fork.

To serve, garnish with cilantro.

Salmon w/ Chanterelle Mushrooms

Yields: 4 Servings

Total Time: 35 Minutes

Prep Time: 15 Minutes

Cook Time: 20 Minutes

Ingredients

• 4 (8 to 10 ounces each) ivory king salmon steaks, center cut

• ½ pound sliced chanterelle mushrooms, sliced (or you can use porcini mushrooms in the absence of the chanterelles)

• 4 ounces extra virgin olive oil, separated

• 6 ounces white wine

• 16 ounces unsalted organic chicken stock

• ½ tbsp. chopped fresh thyme leaves

• 2 tbsp. minced shallots

• 1 tbsp. Minced garlic

• 3 tbsp. coconut oil, divided

• 1 tbsp. Freshly squeezed lemon juice

• A pinch of sea salt

• A pinch of freshly ground black pepper

• Parsley sprigs and lemon wedges to garnish

Directions

Preheat your grill to medium low.

Brush the fish fillets with 1 ounce of extra virgin olive oil and sprinkle with salt and pepper.

Grill for about 6 minutes per side or until cooked through.

In the meantime, set a sauté pan over high heat and add the remaining oil. Add the mushrooms, sea salt and black pepper and sauté for about 2 minutes or until one side caramelizes.

Remove the pan from heat and turn the mushrooms onto the second side; sprinkle with salt and pepper and continue sautéing until slightly browned. Transfer the mushrooms to a strainer and strain off excess oil.

Return the pan to heat and add 1 tablespoon coconut oil; add garlic and shallots and cook until blended. Add thyme and remove from heat. Deglaze with wine and return the pan to heat. Cook until the liquid is reduced to half.

Add the chicken stock and continue cooking until reduced to sauce consistency.

Return the mushrooms to the pan and add the remaining coconut oil. Adjust salt and pepper and add lemon juice.

Place the fish to a serving platter and top with the mushroom mixture; garnish with parsley and lemons to serve.

India Curried Shrimp

Yields: 2 Servings

Total Time: 30 Minutes

Prep Time: 15 Minutes

Cook Time: 15 Minutes

Ingredients

- 8 oz. medium peeled shrimp
- 4 fresh tomatoes, pureed
- 1 medium finely chopped onion
- 2 garlic cloves, minced
- 4 tbsp. extra virgin olive oil
- ½ tsp. turmeric
- ½ tsp. coriander
- ½ tsp. cumin
- 2 tsp. fresh ginger, minced
- 2 tbsp. freshly squeezed lime juice

Direction

Heat oil in a saucepan set over medium heat; sauté onion and garlic until tender. Stir in tomatoes and spices and cook for about 5 minutes. Add shrimp to the simmering mixture and cook for about 10 minutes or until cooked through.

Remove the pan from heat and drizzle with lime juice.

North Shore Baked Salmon File

Yields: 4 Servings

Total Time: 35 Minutes

Prep Time: 15 Minutes

Cook Time: 20 Minutes

Ingredients

- 1 lb. salmon filet
- 1 lemon, thinly sliced
- ½ yellow onion, thinly sliced
- ½ cup white wine
- 1 tsp. minced garlic
- 1 tsp. oregano
- 1 tsp. paprika
- 1 tsp. turmeric

Directions

Preheat your oven to 375°F.

Rinse the fish and place in a 9x13 in baking dish. Add wine and sprinkle with spices. Top with onions and lemon slices and cover with foil.

Bake for about 45 minutes or until fish is cooked through.

Grilled Cod with Spicy Citrus Marinade

Yields: 4 Servings

Total Time:
35 Minutes

Prep Time: 15 Minutes

Cook Time: 20 Minutes

Ingredients

- 1 lb. cod filets
- 2 tbsp. extra virgin olive oil
- 2 minced garlic cloves
- 1/8 tsp. cayenne pepper
- 3 tbsp. freshly squeezed lime juice
- 1 ½ tsp. freshly squeezed lemon juice
- ¼ cup freshly squeezed orange juice
- 1/3 cup water
- 1 tbsp. finely chopped fresh thyme
- 2 tbsp. finely chopped fresh chives

Direction

In a bowl, mix together lemon, lime juice, orange, cayenne pepper, extra virgin olive oil, garlic and water.

Place fish in a dish and add the marinade, reserving ¼ cup; marinate in the refrigerator for at least 30 minutes.

Broil or grill the marinated fish for about 4 minutes per side, basting regularly with the marinade.

Serve the grilled fish on a plate and top with the reserved marinade, thyme and chives.

White Fish with Mushroom Sauce

Yields: 4 Servings

Total Time: 35 Minutes

Prep Time: 15 Minutes

Cook Time: 20 Minutes

Ingredients

- 2 serves fish fillets
- 2 tsp. arrow root
- 1 cup mushrooms, sliced
- 1 clove garlic, finely chopped
- 1 small onion, thinly sliced
- 2 tbsp. extra virgin olive oil
- ½ cup fresh parsley, roughly chopped
- 1 tsp. thyme leaves, finely chopped
- ½ cup water
- A pinch of freshly ground black pepper
- A pinch of sea salt

Directions

Preheat your oven to 350°F.

Add extra virgin olive oil to a frying pan set over medium heat; sauté onion, garlic and mushrooms for about 4 minutes or until mushrooms are slightly tender.

Stir in arrowroot, sea salt, thyme and pepper and cook for about 1 minute.

Stir in water until thickened; stir in parsley and cook for 1 minute more.

Place the fillets on a baking tray lined with parchment paper; cover the fish with mushroom sauce and bake for about 20 minutes or until the fish is cooked through.

PALEO DINNER RECIPES

Ground Lamb & Zucchini

Yields: 4 Servings

Total Time: 45 Minutes

Prep Time: 15 Minutes

Cook Time: 30 Minutes

Ingredients

*   450g lean ground lamb

*   2 medium (6 to 8 inches each) zucchini, diced

*   1 tbsp. coconut oil

*   1-2 cloves garlic, minced

*   2 medium tomatoes, diced

*   2 tbsp. dried oregano

*   1/2 yellow onion, diced

Directions

Rinse and prepare the veggies.

Set a large skillet over medium high heat and add coconut oil when hot; stir in onions and sauté for about 4 minutes or until translucent.

Roll ground lamb into small balls and add to the pan along with oregano and garlic; cook for about 5 minutes. Add tomatoes and zucchini and continue cooking until tender.

Serve and enjoy!

Roasted Beets w/ Balsamic Glaze

Yields: 4 Servings

Total Time: 75 Minutes

Prep Time: 15 Minutes

Cook Time: 60 Minutes

Ingredients

*   5-6 beets (about 3 to 4 inches each)

*   2 tbsp. extra virgin olive oil

*   ¼ tsp. freshly ground black pepper

*   ¼ tsp. sea salt

Directions

Preheat your oven to 325°F.

Rinse and slice beets into quarters; slice each quarter into ¼-inch slices and place them on a baking sheet. Drizzle with extra virgin olive oil and sprinkle with sea salt and pepper; mix well and spread the beets out on the sheet.

Roast for about 60 minutes.

In the meantime, combine maple syrup and vinegar in a pan set over high heat; cook for a few minutes or until the mixture has reduced to a syrup consistency.

Remove the pan from heat and set aside.

When the beets are ready, drizzle with the glaze and sprinkle with orange zest to serve.

Turkey Lettuce Wraps

Yields: 4 Servings

Total Time: 35 Minutes

Prep Time: 15 Minutes

Cook Time: 20 Minutes

Ingredients

* 250g ground turkey

* 1/2 small onion, finely chopped

* 1 garlic clove, minced

* 2 tbsp. extra virgin olive oil

* 1 head lettuce

* 1 tsp. cumin

* 1/2 tbsp. fresh ginger, sliced

* 2 tbsp. freshly squeezed lime juice

* 1-2 tbsp. freshly chopped cilantro

* 1 tsp. freshly ground black pepper

* 1 tsp. sea salt

Directions

Sauté garlic and onion in extra virgin olive oil until fragrant and translucent.

Add turkey and cook well.

Stir in the remaining ingredients and continue cooking for 5 minutes more.

To serve, ladle a spoonful of turkey mixture onto a lettuce leaf and wrap. Enjoy!

Gingery Chicken & Veggies

Yields: 4 Servings

Total Time: 15 Minutes

Prep Time: 10 Minutes

Cook Time: 5 Minutes

Ingredients

- 2 cup skinless, boneless, and cooked chicken breast meat, diced

- ¼ cup extra virgin olive and canola oil mixture

- 1 tsp. powdered ginger

- ½ red onion, sliced

- 2 cloves garlic, minced

- ½ bell pepper, sliced

- 1 cup thinly sliced carrots

- ½ cup finely chopped celery

- 1 cup chicken broth (not salted)

Directions

Add the oil mixture to a skillet set over medium heat; sauté onion and garlic until translucent. Stir in the remaining ingredients and simmer for a few minutes or until the veggies are tender.

Moroccan Chicken Casserole

Yields: 4 Servings

Total Time: 1 Hour 25 Minutes

Prep Time: 10 Minutes

Cook Time: 1 Hour 15 Minutes

Ingredients

- 2-3 pounds of chicken
- 1 head cauliflower
- 3 carrots, peeled and diced
- 2 garlic cloves, finely chopped
- 2 tbsp. finely grated or chopped ginger root
- 1 onion, finely chopped
- 2 tbsp. coconut oil
- 1/2 cup minced cilantro or parsley
- 1 (28-ounce) can diced tomatoes, undrained
- 1 red pepper, cut into thin strips
- 1/2 tsp. cinnamon
- 1/2 tsp. turmeric
- 1 tsp. coriander
- 1 tsp. paprika
- 2 tsp. cumin
- 2 tsp. sea salt
- 1/4 tsp. cayenne, optional, for an extra spicy dish
- 1 medium fresh lemon

Directions

Preheat your oven to 375°F.

Chop cauliflower into small pieces and grate them by pushing them through a processor using a grating blade; evenly spread cauliflower out in a rectangular baking pan.

Sprinkle the chicken with sea salt and black pepper.

Melt 1 tablespoon of coconut oil in a deep pan set over high heat; brown the chicken, for about 5 minutes per side.

Transfer the chicken to a plate and set aside.

Reduce heat to medium and stir in carrots, garlic, ginger and onion; cook for a few minutes or until onion is translucent. Stir in the remaining coconut oil and spices and stir to mix well.

Stir in minced parsley, tomatoes, red pepper and salt and return the chicken. Simmer for about 5 minutes.

Top cauliflower with the chicken mixture and mix well. Arrange lemon slices over the casserole and cover the baking pan with foil; bake for about 35 minutes. Remove the foil and continue baking for 25 minutes more. Serve warm.

Asian Mince Curry

Yields: 4 Servings

Total Time: 1 Hour 10 Minutes

Prep Time: 10 Minutes

Cook Time: 1 Hour

Ingredients

- 450g mince meat
- 4 tbsp. Biriyani curry paste (a mix of sea salt, rampe, curry leaves, tomatoes, nutmeg, cloves, cardamoms, extra virgin olive oil, ginger,
- Garlic, coriander)
- 1 (14.5 oz.) diced tomatoes
- 2 cups diced eggplant
- 4 cups thinly sliced cabbage
- 1 (14.5 oz.) can green peas or 1½ cup fresh
- 1 tbsp. extra virgin olive oil
- 3 garlic cloves, finely chopped
- 1 onion, finely chopped

Directions

Sauté garlic and onion in oil over medium heat until golden brown.

Transfer onion and garlic to a plate and add minced meat to the pan; cook, stirring, until there are no big lumps.

Return the onion and garlic along with green peas, eggplant, cabbage and curry paste; stir until heated through. Stir in diced tomatoes and simmer for about 45 minutes or until the veggies are tender and cooked.

Fried Chili Beef w/ Cashews

Yields: 4 Servings

Total Time: 35 Minutes

Prep Time: 10 Minutes

Cook Time: 25 Minutes

Ingredients

- ½ tbsp. extra virgin olive oil or canola oil
- 1 pound sliced lean beef
- 2 tbsp. freshly squeezed lime juice
- 2 tsp. fish sauce
- 2 tsp. red curry paste
- 1 cup green capsicum, diced
- 24 cashews
- 1 tsp. arrowroot
- 1 tsp. honey
- ½ cup water

Directions

Add oil to a pan set over medium heat; add beef and fry until its no longer pink inside. Stir in red curry paste and cook for a few more minutes.

Stir in honey, lime juice, fish sauce, capsicum and water; simmer for about 10 minutes.

Mix cooked arrowroot with water to make a paste; stir the paste into the sauce to thicken it.

Remove the pan from heat and add the fried cashews. Serve.

Coconut-Crusted Cod

Yields: 4 Servings

Total Time: 35 Minutes

Prep Time: 25 Minutes

Cook Time: 10 Minutes

Ingredients:

- 24 ounces cod fillets, sliced into small strips
- 2 tbsp. coconut oil
- 1 cup finely shredded coconut
- 2 cups coconut milk
- 1 ½ cups coconut flour
- ¼ tsp. sea salt
- 1 ½ tsp. ginger powder

Directions

Rinse and debone the fish fillets.

In a bowl, combine ginger powder, coconut flour and sea salt; set aside.

Add coconut milk to another bowl and set aside.

Add shredded coconut to another bowl and set aside.

Dip the fillets into coconut milk, then into the flour mixture, back into the milk, and finally into shredded coconut.

Add coconut oil to a skillet set over high heat; when melted and hot, add the fish fillets and cook for about 5 minutes per side or until cooked through.

Curried Chicken Salad

Yields: 3 to 4 Servings

Total Time: 10 Minutes

Prep Time: 10 Minutes

Cook Time: 0 Minutes

Ingredients:

- ½ cup mashed garlic and avocado, at room temperature
- 1 tsp. apple-cider vinegar
- ½ lemon, juiced
- 2 tsp. powdered turmeric
- 1 tsp. powdered ginger
- ¼ tsp. sea salt
- 1 lb. shredded pastured chicken breast
- ¼ cup chopped red onion
- ¼ cup raisins
- 2 tbsp. chopped parsley

Directions

In a bowl, mix together lemon juice, apple cider vinegar, avocado mash, ginger, turmeric and sea salt until well blended.

Add chicken breasts, raisins, and red onion; stir to mix well.

Garnish with chopped parsley and serve.

Mexican Chicken Served With 'Rice'

Yields: 3 Servings

Total Time: 45 Minutes

Prep Time: 10 Minutes

Cook Time: 30 Minutes

Ingredients

•	1 pound boneless and skinless grilled chicken breast, diced into small pieces

•	1 medium avocado

•	4 tbsp. Extra virgin olive oil

•	1 can (4 ounce) diced green chilies

•	1 head cauliflower, trimmed

•	1 cup celery, finely diced

•	1 medium onion, diced

•	A pinch of chili powder, ground cumin and oregano and to taste

•	1 tsp. sea salt

•	Salsa, optional

Directions

Heat extra virgin olive oil in a skillet set over medium heat. Add onion and sauté for about 10 minutes or until tender.

Add celery and sauté for 5 minutes more.

Process cauliflower in a food processor until you achieve the texture of rice.

Stir cauliflower in the onion mixture and cook, covered, for about 10 minutes or until tender.

Add chicken, chilies, chili powder, oregano, cumin, and sea salt.

Serve topped with salsa and avocado.

Asian Stir Fry

Yields: 4 Servings

Total Time: 45 Minutes

Prep Time: 10 Minutes

Cook Time: 30 Minutes

Ingredients

- 2 tbsp. coconut oil

- 1 pound boneless, skinless chicken breast

- 1 tbsp. honey

- 2 tbsp. Vinegar

- 2 tbsp. toasted sesame oil

- 2 tbsp. arrowroot powder

- 1 cup sliced zucchini (about 1 small zucchini)

- 4 ounces stemmed and thinly sliced shiitake mushrooms (about 1 cup)

- 1 ½ cups sliced strips of baby bock choy

- 1 cup thinly sliced carrots

- 4 cups sliced broccoli

- 1 cup finely chopped onion

- ½ tsp. Sea salt

- 1½ cups water

Directions

Rinse and pat dry the chicken; cut into small cubes and place them on a plate.

Add coconut oil to a skillet set over medium heat to melt.

Add onion and sauté for about 10 minutes or until tender and translucent.

Add zucchini, mushrooms, bock choy, and sea salt; sauté for about 5 minutes.

Stir in a cup of water and cook, covered, for about 10 minutes or until veggies are wilted.

Dissolve arrowroot powder in a bowl with ½ cup of water, stirring until well blended.

Stir the arrowroot mixture into the veggies and continue cooking for 3 minutes more or until the sauce is thick and glossy.

Stir in honey, sesame oil and vinegar. Serve hot.

Zucchini Noodles

Yields: 2 to 4 Servings

Total Time: 25 Minutes

Prep Time: 10 Minutes

Cook Time: 15 Minutes

Ingredients

- 1 tbsp. extra virgin olive oil

- 1 pound zucchini

- 1 tsp. spice mix

Directions

Heat extra virgin olive oil in a large sauté pan

Add zucchini noodles; stir in the seasoning and cook for about 5 minutes or until noodles are tender

Serve.

Spiced Chicken w/ Grilled Lime

Yields: 4 Servings

Total Time: 50 Minutes

Prep Time: 10 Minutes

Cook Time: 40 Minutes

Ingredients

- 3 pounds bone-in chicken pieces
- 1 tbsp. garlic powder
- 1 tbsp. smoked paprika
- 2 tbsp. coconut sugar
- 6 limes, halved
- 1 tsp. allspice
- 1 tbsp. Freshly squeezed ground black pepper
- ½ tsp. sea salt

Directions

Place limes and chicken pieces in a bowl.

In a small bowl, mix together garlic powder, paprika, coconut sugar, allspice, pepper and salt; pour over the chicken and mix well.

Grill the chicken and limes over medium heat for about 20 minutes per side. Serve.

Turkey Hash

Yields: 4 Servings

Total Time: 40 Minutes

Prep Time: 10 Minutes

Cook Time: 30 Minutes

Ingredients

• 2 cups turkey, diced

• 3 cups pumpkin or butternut squash, peeled and sliced into small cubes

• 1 large onion, diced

• 2 tbsp. extra virgin olive oil

• 1 cup water

• ¼ tsp. freshly ground black pepper

• ½ tsp. sea salt

Directions

Add extra virgin olive oil to a large skillet set over medium heat; add onion and sauté for about 10 minutes, stirring, or until caramelized.

Add pumpkin or squash and cook, covered, for about 10 minutes

Add the turkey, sea salt and pepper and continue cooking for about 10 minutes.

Serve hot.

Sesame Salmon Burgers

Yields: 12 burgers

Total Time: 37 Minutes

Prep Time: 25 Minutes

Cook Time: 12 Minutes

Ingredients

- 1 pound salmon, skin removed
- 1 tbsp. coconut flour
- 2 large free range eggs
- ¼ cup toasted sesame seeds
- ¼ cup finely chopped scallions (only green and white parts)
- 1 tsp. fresh ginger, peeled and minced
- 1 clove garlic, pressed
- 1 tbsp. Ume plum vinegar
- 1 tbsp. toasted sesame oil
- Coconut oil, for frying

Directions

Rinse the fish and pat dry with paper towel; cut into ¼-inch cubes.

Mix together eggs, sesame seeds, scallions, ginger, garlic, Ume, oil, and salmon in a large bowl.

Stir in the coconut flour and form small patties.

Add coconut oil to a skillet set over medium high heat to melt. Add the patties and cook for about 6 minutes per side or until golden brown.

Place the cooked patties onto a plate lined with paper towel to serve.

Grilled Lemony Chicken

Yields: 2 Servings

Total Time: 6 Hours 25 Minutes

Prep Time: 6 Hours 15 Minutes

Cook Time: 10 Minutes

Ingredients

- 1 pound boneless and skinless chicken breasts, halved
- 1 ½ tsp. freshly minced thyme leaves
- ½ tsp. freshly ground black pepper
- ⅓ cup extra virgin olive oil
- ⅓ cup lemon juice, freshly squeezed
- 1 tsp. sea salt
- 2 large carrots, julienned or grated
- 1 head Romaine lettuce, bottom chiffonade leaves removed
- Nut Sauce

Directions

Whisk together extra virgin olive oil, lemon juice, thyme, sea salt and pepper in a bowl to make the marinade.

Place chicken in a baking dish; pour the marinade over the chicken and marinate in the refrigerator for at least 6 hours.

When ready, heat your grill and grill the chicken for about 10 minutes per side or until cooked through.

Remove from oven, let cool and cut into small slices.

To serve, place romaine on a platter and top with carrots; place the grilled chicken over the veggies and serve with the nut sauce.

Barbecued salmon with lemon and herbs

Yields: 12 Servings

Total Time: 4 Hours 27 Minutes

Prep Time: 4 Hours 15 Minutes

Cook Time: 12 Minutes

Ingredients

*   12 (180 grams each) Atlantic salmon fillets, with skin on
*   1/2 cup extra virgin olive oil
*   1 bunch roughly chopped lemon thyme
*   1/3 cup finely chopped dill leaves
*   2 tbsp. drained and chopped capers
*   2 fresh lemons, juiced
*   2 garlic cloves, finely chopped
*   A pinch of sea salt
*   Lemon wedges, to garnish

Directions

In a large jug, mix together lemon thyme, dill, capers, 1/3 cup lemon juice, garlic, extra virgin olive oil, sea salt and pepper.

Arrange salmon fillets, in a single layer, in a ceramic dish and pour over half of the marinade. Turn it over and pour over the remaining marinade. Refrigerate, covered, for about 4 hours.

Remove the fish from the refrigerator at least 30 minutes before cooking.

Grease barbecue plate and heat on medium high. Barbecue the marinated fish, skin side down, for about 3 minutes. Turn and continue barbecuing, basting occasionally with the marinade, for 6 minutes more or until cooked through.

Serve garnished with lemon wedges.

Fish with Herb sauce

Yields: 4 Servings

Total Time: 30 Minutes

Prep Time: 15 Minutes

Cook Time: 15 Minutes

Ingredients

• 4 (180 grams each) white fish fillets (such as snapper or blue-eye), with skin on

• 1/3 cup extra virgin olive oil

• 1 cup roughly torn flat-leaf parsley leaves

• 3 garlic cloves, sliced

• 1 large fresh lemon

• 1/4 cup oregano leaves

• 12 basil leaves, torn

• 12 mint leaves, torn

• Crusty bread, to serve

Directions

Preheat your oven to 350°F.

Peel the lemon and squeeze out the juice into a bowl; stir in extra virgin olive oil, herbs, garlic, and season. Set aside.

Add the remaining oil to an ovenproof pan set over medium high heat; stir in lemon rind for about 30 seconds. Place the seasoned fish in the pan, skin side down and cook for about 4 minutes or until crisp.

Transfer the pan to the oven and cook for about 5 minutes or until the fish is cooked through.

Remove the pan from the oven and transfer to low heat; pour over the herb mixture and cook until just warmed through. Serve with crusty bread.

Roasted Seafood w/ Herbs &Lemon

Yields: 4 Servings

Total Time: 25 Minutes

Prep Time: 15 Minutes

Cook Time: 10 Minutes

Ingredients

*   1/4 cup extra virgin olive oil

*   8 scallops on the half shell

*   8 large green prawns

*   8 scampi, halved and cleaned

*   2 garlic cloves, finely chopped

*   2 tbsp. chopped flat-leaf parsley

*   Finely grated lemon zest

*   Freshly squeezed lemon juice from 1 lemon

*   2 tbsp. finely chopped lemon thyme

Directions

Preheat your oven to 400°F.

Arrange the seafood in a single layer in a baking dish.

Combine together lemon juice, zest, garlic, extra virgin olive oil, and thyme; brush over the seafood and season well.

Bake in the preheated oven for about 10 minutes or until cooked through.

Sprinkle with chopped parsley and serve garnished with lemon wedges.

Cucumber & Avocado Salad

Yields: 16 Servings

Total Time: 22 Minutes

Prep Time: 10 Minutes

Cook Time: 0 Minutes

Ingredients

- 1/4 cup extra virgin olive oil
- 1/4 cup lemon juice
- 175g baby salad leaves
- 2 thinly sliced Lebanese cucumbers
- 4 green onions, thinly sliced
- 2 medium avocados, chopped

Directions

In a bowl, combine together salad leaves, cucumber, onion, and avocado.

Mix together extra virgin olive oil and lemon juice in a jar and season with sea salt. Shake to mix well and pour over the salad to serve.

Paprika and chili kale chips

Yields: 4 Servings

Total Time: 22 Minutes

Prep Time: 10 Minutes

Cook Time: 12Minutes

Ingredients

- 2 tbsp. extra virgin olive oil
- 1 bunch curly kale
- 1/2 tsp. dried red chili flakes
- 1 tsp. paprika
- A pinch of sea salt

Directions

Preheat your oven to 350°F.

Prepare two baking trays by lining them with baking papers.

Trim the center stems from kale and cop into small pieces.

In a large bowl, mix together chili, paprika, and extra virgin olive oil; add the kale and toss until well coated.

Spread the kale out on the prepared baking dishes and bake for about 15 minutes or until kale is crisp.

Sprinkle with sea salt to serve.

PALEO SNACKS

Chicken Liver Pâté

Yields: 2 Servings

Total Time: 5 Minutes

Prep Time: 5 Minutes

Cook Time: 0 Minutes

Ingredients

• 1/2 lb. chicken livers

• 3 thin slices bacon, chopped in cubes (if strictly not paleo)

• 1 clove garlic, minced

• 3 tbsp. sherry or apple cider vinegar

• 4 tbsp. chopped parsley

• 1 large onion, diced

• 3/4 cup coconut oil

• A pinch of sea salt

• A pinch of freshly ground black pepper

• Fresh nutmeg, if desired

Directions

Set a large pan over medium high heat; add bacon and cook for about 3 minutes. Stir in garlic, onion and ¼ cup coconut oil and cook for 4 minutes more.

Cut out the white parts of the leaves and add them to the pot.

Continue cooking for about 10 minutes or until cooked through.

Stir in sherry, pepper, parsley, nutmeg, sea salt and pepper. Remove the pan from heat and transfer the mixture to a food processor or blender; process until very smooth. Transfer to a serving dish.

Melt the remaining coconut milk and evenly pour over the pâté.

Refrigerate, covered, until it hardens. Enjoy as a snack on lettuce leaves, on celery sticks or as is.

Easy Guacamole

Yields: 2 ½ cups of Guacamole

Total Time: 5 Minutes

Prep Time: 5 Minutes

Cook Time: 0 Minutes

Ingredients

- 3 medium avocados or 4 small ones
- 2 tbsp. freshly squeezed lemon or lime juice
- 1/2 cup chopped cilantro
- 1/2 white onion
- 1 firm tomato, finely diced
- A pinch of sea salt
- A pinch of freshly ground black pepper

Directions

Cut the avocados into halves and scoop out the flesh into a large bowl.

Using a fork, mash the avocado until smooth.

Stir in the other ingredients and enjoy right away.

Baked Cinnamon Apple Chips

Yields: 2 Servings

Total Time: 2 Hours 5 Minutes

Prep Time: 5 Minutes

Cook Time: 2 Hours

Ingredients

•	1-2 apples

•	1 tsp. cinnamon

Directions

Preheat your oven to 200°F.

Slice the apples thinly with a mandolin or sharp knife. Discard the seeds.

Line baking sheet with parchment paper and arrange on the apple slices in a single layer.

Sprinkle with cinnamon and bake for about 1 hour; flip them over and continue baking for 1 hour more, flipping occasionally, until crispy.

Store the apple chips in an airtight container.

Zucchini Ribbon Salad

Zucchini ribbons are barely slicked with olive oil and lemon juice to make a great dinner dish. This recipe is simple and easy to make and requires no fancy gadget to get it ready.

Yield: 4 Servings

Total Time: 15 Minutes

Prep Time: 15 Minutes

Cook Time: 0 Minutes

Ingredients

- 300g zucchini

- 2 tbsp. olive oil

- Juice of 1 lemon

- ½ small pack mint, chopped

- ½ small pack chives, chopped

Directions

Combine lemon juice, salt and pepper in a bowl. Whisk in extra virgin olive oil and then stir in the chopped herbs.

Spiralis the zucchini through a spiralizer into the bowl with the dressing. Toss to combine well and serve immediately.

Roasted Sweet Potato Chips

Yields: 1 to 2 Servings

Total Time: 1 Hour 15 Minutes

Prep Time: 15 Minutes

Cook Time: 1 Hour

Ingredients

- 1 tbsp. extra virgin olive oil

- 1 large sweet potato

- Salt

Directions

Preheat your oven to 300°F.

Scrub potato and slice into thin slices.

Toss together the potato slices with salt and extra virgin olive oil in a bowl; arrange them in a single layer on a cookie sheet. Bake for about 1 hour, flipping every 15 minutes, until crispy and browned.

Roasted Asparagus

Yield: 4 Servings

Total Time: 15 Minutes

Prep Time: 5 Minutes

Cook Time: 10 Minutes

Ingredients

*   1 tbsp. extra virgin olive oil

*   1 pound fresh asparagus

*   1 medium lemon, zested

*   1/2 tsp. freshly grated nutmeg

*   1/2 tsp. kosher salt

*   ½ tsp. black pepper

Directions

Preheat your oven to 500°F. Arrange asparagus on an aluminum foil and drizzle with extra virgin olive oil; toss until well coated. Spread the asparagus in a single layer and fold the edges of foil to make a tray. Roast the asparagus in the oven for about 5 minutes; toss and continue roasting for 5 minutes more or until browned. Sprinkle the roasted asparagus with nutmeg, salt, zest and pepper to serve.

Guacamole w/ Vegetables

Yields: 2 Servings

Total Time: 15 Minutes

Prep Time: 15 Minutes

Cook Time: 0 Minutes

Ingredients

- 2 avocados
- Juice of 1 lime
- Zest of lime
- 1 clove garlic, peeled, minced
- 1/4 red onion, peeled, diced
- Fresh cilantro, chopped
- Sea salt
- Veggies (peppers, celery, cucumber etc.) for serving

Directions

In a bowl, mash together all ingredients to your desired consistency. Garnish with cilantro sprigs and store, covered, in a plastic wrap.

Kale Chips

Extra virgin olive oil, nutritious yeast and salt are all you need to turn the fresh kale into delicious and nutritious snacks. They are crunchy and addictive.

Yields: 6 Servings

Total Time: 35 Minutes

Prep Time: 15 Minutes

Cook Time: 20 Minutes

Ingredients

- 6 ounces kale

- 1 tbsp. extra virgin olive oil

- 2 tbsp. nutritional yeast

- Sea salt

Directions

Preheat your oven to 300°F.

Wash and pat dry kale, and then remove tough center ribs and stems; cut into large pieces.

In a large bowl, toss together the chopped kale with extra virgin olive oil and sea salt; arrange the leaves in a single layer on a baking sheet and bake until crisp, for about 20 minutes. Transfer the baking sheet to rack to cool the kale chips before serving.

Hard-Boiled Eggs w/ Avocado

Yields: 2 Servings

Total Time: 15 Minutes

Prep Time: 15 Minutes

Cook Time: 0 Minutes

Ingredients

- 1/2 avocado, diced

- 1 tsp. fresh herbs

- 2 hard-boiled free range eggs

- Dash of hot sauce

Directions

Peel the eggs and rinse under cold water. Slice the eggs into quarters and combine with diced avocado in a bowl. Garnish with fresh herbs and hot sauce and enjoy!

Healthy F*ried Plantain*

Yields: 2 Servings

Total Time: 28 Minutes

Prep Time: 10 Minutes

Cook Time: 18 Minutes

Ingredients

- 2 very ripe plantains
- 1 tsp. ground cinnamon
- 1/4 cup water
- 3 tbsp. virgin coconut oil

Directions

Cut the peeled plantains in half; again cut the halves into half lengthwise.

Add coconut oil to a pan set over medium high heat; sauté the plantains for about 8 minutes. Turn them over and add enough water to cover; simmer for about 10 minutes or until softened.

Sprinkle with cinnamon and serve warm.

Pickled Veggies

Yields: 16 Servings

Total Time: 17 Minutes

Prep Time: 15 Minutes

Cook Time: 2 Minutes

Ingredients:

- 1 ½ cups green beans, halved
- 2 cups sliced zucchini
- 1 ½ cups sliced onions
- 1 large red pepper, sliced
- 1 tbsp. honey
- 1 tbsp. pickling spice
- 1 cup apple cider vinegar
- Salt

Directions:

Lightly sprinkle salt over onions, beans, zucchini and pepper; let stand for at least 15 minutes. Rinse well and stir into boiling water; cook for about 2 minutes. Drain and rinse with cold water.

Combine pickling spice ad vinegar in a pan; bring to a gentle boil; remove from heat and let cool. Stir in honey and pour over the veggies. You can refrigerate up to 14 days.

Stuffed Celery Bites

Yields: 8 Servings

Total Time: 19 Minutes

Prep Time: 15 Minutes

Cook Time: 4 Minutes

Ingredients:

- Celery leaves
- 2 tbsp. Sunflower seeds, dry-roasted
- 1/4 cup Italian cheese blend, shredded
- 1 (8-ounce) fat-free cream cheese
- 8 stalks celery
- 1 clove garlic, minced
- 2 tbsp. pine nuts
- Olive oil cooking spray

Directions:

Coat a nonstick skillet with olive oil cooking spray; add garlic and pine nuts and sauté over medium heat for about 4 minutes or until the nuts are golden brown. Set aside.

Cut off the wide base and tops from celery and remove 2 thin strips from the round side of celery to create a flat surface.

Combine Italian cheese and cream cheese in a bowl; spread into celery and cut each celery stalk into 2-inch pieces.

Sprinkle half of the celery pieces with sunflower seeds and half with the pine nut mixture; cover and let stand for at least 4 hours before serving.

Pesto-Stuffed Mushrooms

Yields: 14 Servings

Total Time: 4 Hours 15 Minutes

Prep Time: 4 Hour 15 Minutes

Cook Time: 0 Minutes

Ingredients:

*   14+ button mushrooms, washed and stemmed

*   1/2 cup extra virgin olive oil

*   3 cloves garlic

*   2 cups basil

*   1/2 cup pine nuts

*   1 cup walnuts

*   1/2 tsp. sea salt

Directions:

Arrange the mushroom caps top-side down on a plate.

In a food processor, blend together stuffing ingredients until very smooth.

Scoop an equal amount of the stuffing into each cap and dehydrate at 105°F until soft, for about 6 hours.

Serve warm.

Healthy Sautéed Kale

Yields: 4 Servings

Total Time: 30 Minutes

Prep Time: 10 Minutes

Cook Time: 20 Minutes

Ingredients

- 1 bunch kale, chopped
- 1 medium onion, chopped
- 2 tbsp. extra virgin olive oil
- ¼ tsp. Sea salt

Directions

Heat extra virgin olive oil in a pan set over medium heat. Stir in onion and sauté over medium low heat for about 15 minutes or until caramelized.

Stir in kale and sauté for 5 more minutes. Season with salt to serve.

Vinegar & Salt Kale Chips

Kale seasoned with apple cider vinegar is a deluxe combination. These kale chips are a crowd pleaser!

Yields: 4 Servings

Total Time: 37 Minutes

Prep Time: 25 Minutes

Cook Time: 12 Minutes

Ingredients

- 1 tsp. Extra virgin olive oil
- 1 head kale, chopped
- 1 tbsp. apple cider vinegar
- ½ tsp. sea salt

Directions

Place kale in a bowl and drizzle with vinegar and extra virgin olive oil; sprinkle with salt and massage the ingredients with hands.

Spread the kale out onto two paper-lined baking sheets and bake at 375°F for about 12 minutes or until crispy.

Let cool for about 10 minutes before serving.

Squash Fries

Yields: 6 Servings

Total Time: 25 Minutes

Prep Time: 15 Minutes

Cook Time: 10 Minutes

Ingredients

- 1 tbsp. grapeseed oil

- 1 medium butternut squash

- 1/8 tsp. Sea salt

Directions

Peel and remove seeds from the squash; cut into thin slices and place them in a bowl. Coat with extra virgin olive oil and grapeseed oil; sprinkle with salt and toss to coat well.

Arrange the squash slices onto three baking sheets and broil in the oven until crispy.

Spinach Cake

Make this delicious spinach cake with those pounds of spinach crowding in the vegetable drawer of your fridge. It's fluffy, moist and irresistible.

Yields: 12 Spinach Cakes

Total Time: 1 Hour Minutes

Prep Time: 15 Minutes

Cook Time: 45 Minutes

Ingredients

- 1 ½ pounds spinach, rinsed
- 2 large eggs, whisked
- 2 cloves garlic, minced
- 1 cup pine nuts
- 3 tbsp. grapeseed oil
- ½ cup currants
- 1 tsp. sea salt

Directions

Wilt spinach in a pan set over low heat for about 5 minutes; drain and let cool a bit before squeezing moisture out of the spinach.

Pulse the spinach in a food processor until coarsely chopped; set aside.

Warm oil in a skillet; add pine nuts and sauté for a few minutes or until golden browned.

Stir in garlic and continue cooking for 1 more minute.

Combine the pine mixture, currants, blended spinach and salt in a bowl; spread the mixture into a coated baking dish and bake at 350°F for about 35 minutes.

Carrot French Fries

Turn carrots into fun fries with a healthier profile by baking then in the oven and serving them fry-style. It is a healthy way to make kids eat veggies.

Yields: 2 Servings

Total Time: 35 Minutes

Prep Time: 15 Minutes

Cook Time: 20 Minutes

Ingredients

- 2 tbsp. extra virgin olive oil

- 6 large carrots

- ½ tsp. sea salt

Directions

Chop the carrots into 2-inch sections and then cut each section into thin sticks.

Toss together the carrots sticks with extra virgin olive oil and salt in a bowl and spread into a baking sheet lined with parchment paper.

Bake the carrot sticks at 425F° for about 20 minutes or until browned.

Roasted Balsamic Beets

Yields: 4 Servings

Total Time: 1 Hour 30 Minutes

Prep Time: 15 Minutes

Cook Time: 1 Hour 15 Minutes

Ingredients

- 2 tbsp. extra virgin olive oil

- 1 tbsp. balsamic vinegar

- 3-4 medium beets

- ½ tsp. sea salt

Directions

Scrub the beets and wash well; cut into 6 wedges and place them in a baking dish.

Drizzle the beets with extra virgin olive oil, vinegar and salt and bake, covered, at 375°F for about 1 hour. Uncover and continue baking for 15 more minutes or until almost tender.

Candied Macadamia Nuts

These are perfect healthy appetizer, snack or desserts.

Yields: 6 Servings

Total Time: 30 Minutes

Prep Time: 15 Minutes

Cook Time: 15 Minutes

Ingredients

- 2 cups macadamia nuts
- 1 tbsp. extra virgin olive oil
- 2 tbsp. Honey
- ½ tsp. sea salt

Directions

In a bowl, toss together all ingredients and spread into a baking dish. Bake at 350°F for about 15 minutes or until browned.

Remove from oven and let cool before serving.

Fig Tapenade

The clever mix of Kalamata olives, figs, and olive oil makes this fig tapenade very special and healthy.

Yields: 16 Servings

Total Time: 15 Minutes

Prep Time: 15 Minutes

Cook Time: 0 Minutes

Ingredients

- 1 cup dried figs

- ½ tsp. balsamic vinegar

- 1 tbsp. extra virgin olive oil

- 1 cup Kalamata olives

- 1 tbsp. chopped fresh thyme

- ½ cup water

Directions

Pulse the figs in a food processor until well chopped; add water and continue pulsing to form a paste. Add olives and pulse until well blended.

Add thyme, vinegar and extra virgin olive oil and pulse until very smooth. Serve with walnut crackers.

Veggie Snack

Yields: 1 Serving

Total Time: 10 Minutes

Prep Time: 10 Minutes

Cook Time: 0 Minutes

Ingredients

- 1 yellow pepper
- 5 stalks celery
- 5 carrots

Directions

Scrub the carrots and rinse under running water.

Rinse celery and yellow pepper; deseed the pepper and chop the veggies into small sticks.

Combine in a bowl and serve.

Guacamole Deviled Eggs

For parties and potlucks, these tasty guacamole deviled egg are a simple, healthy hit!

Yields: 12 Servings

Total Time: 40 Minutes

Prep Time: 40 Minutes

Cook Time: 0 Minutes

Ingredients

- 2 ripe avocados
- 6 large hard-boiled eggs, peeled
- 1 tbsp. lime juice
- 1 tbsp. chopped chives
- ¼ cup chopped cilantro
- 1 tsp. red pepper flakes
- ½ tsp. sea salt
- Chili powder, for garnish

Directions

Cut the hard-boiled eggs into two equal parts and scoop out the yolks.

Mash together the egg yolks and avocados in a bowl until smooth. Stir in red pepper flakes, salt, lime juice, chives and cilantro; spoon the filling into the egg whites and refrigerate for at least 30 minutes.

Sprinkle with chili powder to serve.

Curried Roasted Cauliflower

Yield: 4 Servings

Total Time: 37 Minutes

Prep Time: 10 Minutes

Cook Time: 27 Minutes

Ingredients

•   1 large head cauliflower, trimmed and cut into small florets

•   1 cup coconut milk

•   2 tbsp. chopped fresh ginger root

•   2 tbsp. chopped onion

•   1 tbsp. extra virgin olive oil

•   2 tbsp. coconut oil

•   1 tsp. minced garlic

•   ¼ tsp. mustard seeds

•   ¼ tsp. ground cardamom

•   ¼ tsp. ground cumin

•   ¼ tsp. turmeric

•   1 tbsp. curry powder

Directions

Preheat your oven to 400°F. Prepare a 13x 18–inch pan by lining it with parchment paper.

Combine olive oil and coconut oil in a saucepan set over low heat; stir in garlic, ginger and onion and sauté for about 7 minutes or until onion is tender. Stir in coconut milk and simmer for about 5 minutes. Stir in cauliflower, mustard seeds, cardamom, cumin, turmeric, and curry; cook for about 15 minutes or until the liquid has reduced substantially.

Transfer the cauliflower mixture to the prepared pan and bake for about 30 minutes or until golden. Serve warm.

Healthy Spiced Nuts

Yields: 4 Servings

Total Time: 20 Minutes

Prep Time: 10 Minutes

Cook Time: 10 Minutes

Ingredients

- 1 tbsp. extra virgin olive oil
- ⅔ cup walnuts
- ⅔ cup pecans
- ⅔ cup almonds
- ½ tsp. sea salt
- ½ tsp. pepper
- ½ tsp. cumin
- 1 tsp. chili powder

Directions

Put the nuts in a skillet set over medium heat and toast until lightly browned.

In the meantime, prepare the spice mixture; combine black pepper, cumin, chili and salt in a bowl.

Coat the toasted nuts with extra virgin olive oil and sprinkle with the spice mixture to serve.

Sesame Crackers

Yields: 96 Crackers

Total Time: 32 Minutes

Prep Time: 20 Minutes

Cook Time: 12 Minutes

Ingredients

- 1 cup sesame seeds
- 2 tbsp. grapeseed oil
- 2 large free range eggs, beaten
- 1 ½ tsp. sea salt
- 3 cups almond flour, blanched

Directions

Stir together sesame seeds, almond flour, oil, eggs and salt in a large bowl until well combined.

Divide the dough into two portions.

Place each into two baking sheets lined with parchment papers and cover with parchment paper.

Spread the dough between the papers to cover the entire baking sheet and remove the top paper.

With a pizza cutter or knife, cut the dough into 2-inch squares and bake at 350°F until golden brown, for about 12 minutes.

Cool before serving.

PALEO DRINKS

Paleo Almond Milk

Yields: 12 Servings

Prep time: 5 Minutes

Ingredients

- 4 cups water, plus extra for soaking almonds
- 1 cup raw almonds
- 1 tsp. cinnamon
- 1 tsp. vanilla, optional
- 2 tbsp. raw honey, optional

Directions

Soak raw almonds in a large bowl of cold water overnight.

Rinse and drain the soaked almonds.

Transfer to a blender and add 4 cups water and the optional ingredients; blend the mixture on high speed for about 3 minutes or until very smooth.

Strain the mixture through a cheese cloth or a nut milk bag into a pitcher.

(You may dry the nut mixture on a baking sheet to use as almond meal in other recipes).

Chill the almond milk for at least 1 hour.

Paleo Mango lassie

Yields: 4 Servings

Prep Time: 5 Minutes

Ingredients

- 3 tsp. lemon juice
- 3 (50g) medjool dates
- ½ cup (70g) cashews
- 1 medium peeled (140g) banana
- 1 medium peeled, seeded and diced mango (350g)
- 1½ cups ice
- 1 cup water
- pinch salt
- Cardamom or nutmeg to garnish, optional

Directions

Combine together all the ingredients, except nutmeg, in a food processor or blender and pulse at high until very smooth and creamy.

Divide the lassie among the serving glasses; garnish with cardamom or nutmeg and enjoy!

Paleo Strawberry Lemonade

Yields: 6 Servings

Prep Time: 10 Minutes

Ingredients

- 1 pint strawberries, stems removed and rinsed and
- 3/4 - 1 1/4 cup raw honey
- 8 cups water
- 1 1/2 cups lemon juice (from 8-10 lemons)

Directions

Prepare the strawberries and squeeze lemon juice.

Place the strawberries in a blender and blend until very smooth.

Combine together the strawberries, raw honey, 1 cup water, and lemon juice in a saucepan set over medium-high heat; bring the mixture to a gentle boil, stirring to combine well.

Pour the remaining water into a large pitcher and stir in the strawberry-lemon mixture. Taste to see if the lemonade requires any adjustments. If too sour add a little more raw honey and water. If too sweet, add a little more lemon juice and water. If too plain add honey and lemon juice.

Chill for a few hours before serving.

Paleo Antioxidant Berry Shake

Yields: 4 Servings

Prep Time: 5 Minutes

Ingredients

- 1 tbsp. chia seeds
- 1/2 cup frozen blueberries
- 1/2 cup frozen raspberries
- 1/2 frozen banana
- 1/4 cup cold water
- 1/2 cup coconut milk

Directions

Combine together all ingredients in a blender and pulse on high until very smooth. Add more water if needed to attain your desired consistency. Serve immediately.

Cranberry Apple Detox Juice

Yields: 1 big glass (2 servings)

Prep time: 10 minutes

Ingredients

- 1/2 peeled medium lemon
- 1 tsp. grated ginger
- 3 romaine lettuce leaves
- 3 celery stalks
- 1 apple
- 1.5 cups raw cranberries

Directions

Run the ingredients through a juicer and serve immediately.

Berry Delicious

Yields: 4 Servings

Prep Time: 2 Hours 5 Minutes

Ingredients:

- 1 cup lemon juice
- 1 cup fresh mixed berries
- A few freshly chopped mint leaves
- ½ cup raw honey
- 4 cups cold water

Directions

Place berries in a jar and gently crush them apart.

Add lemon juice, mint leaves and raw honey. Add water and stir to combine well.

Refrigerate the drink for at least 2 hours for the flavors to infuse together.

Divide among serving glasses; garnish each glass with a few mint leaves and ice cubes. Enjoy!

Conclusion

Thank you again for downloading this book!

I hope this book was able to help you to lose your weight , stay healthy and learn about the things you need to know in following the Paleo Diet and living the Paleo Life.

The next step is to take action.

Again above is a guideline for you to help get started. Feel free to change the diets according to your desires . If you follow the tips and try the recipes I shared with you , you will definitely see better and a healthier you.

Again thank you for downloading this book . Spread the good news and enjoy the Paleo Life style today!

Finally , if you've received value from this book , please take the time to share your thoughts and post a review on Amazon. It'd be greatly appreciated!

⇨   <u>Click here to leave a review for this book on Amazon!</u>

Thank you and good luck!

Claim Your FREE Bonus!

As a token of appreciation for downloading my book, I would like to give away a FREE BONUS report, "**8 Effective and Helpful Tips of Losing Weight**" Just for you!

May you gain many valuable insights in achieving your weight loss goals!

⇨ <u>CLICK HERE TO CLAIM YOUR FREE BONUS REPORT!</u>

Plus, by signing up to our subscription, you will also receive FREE KINDLE BOOKS, RECIPES, WEIGHT LOSS TIPS AND TOOLS, and MANY MORE to help you attain the weight you desire.

⇨ <u>CLICK HERE TO CLAIM YOUR FREE BONUS REPORT!</u>

See you on the inside!

43673255R00093

Made in the USA
Middletown, DE
15 May 2017